Magdalene House

Magdalene House

A PLACE ABOUT MERCY

Sarah VanHooser Suiter

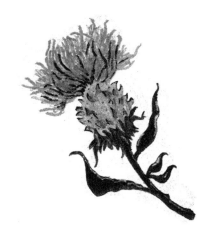

Vanderbilt University Press

Nashville

This book is printed on acid-free paper.
Manufactured in the United States of America

Title page illustration adapted from a painting
by Sandra Binczek, a graduate of Magdalene House.

Library of Congress Cataloging-in-Publication Data on file

ISBN 978-0-8265-1837-8 (printed hardcover)
ISBN 978-0-8265-1838-5 (paperback)
ISBN 978-0-8265-1839-2 (e-book)

LC control number 2011038284
LC classification PT9876.22.A6933 Z78 2012
Dewey class number 839.73/8

In my own particular life, I know better than anybody else the places I've messed up, and I have learned more from mercy than from justice. And I don't think the women at Magdalene were learning anything from the "justice" system. So I wanted this to be a place about mercy.

   —Becca Stevens, Magdalene House founder

CONTENTS

ACKNOWLEDGMENTS

DURING THE COURSE OF writing this book, I have been supported, encouraged, challenged, and loved by too many people to count. This book would not be possible without them, nor would my life be nearly as rich and full. "Thank you" seems an inadequate expression to convey my gratitude, but thanks I offer, wholeheartedly, to the people who have played major roles in helping me tell this story about the Magdalene community.

To residents, graduates, staff, and volunteers of Magdalene House and Thistle Farms, I am humbled and honored to take my place in your circle. Thank you for welcoming me, allowing me to be a part of your lives, and sharing your stories with me. I have found healing, laughter, and creativity among you, and I am truly grateful to call you my friends.

Thank you to Michael Ames, three anonymous reviewers, and a host of wise and intelligent mentors and colleagues, including Craig Anne Heflinger, Joe Cunningham, Paul Dokecki, Melissa Snarr, Beth Shinn, Brooke Ackerly, Bill Partridge, Darcy Freedman, Lyndi Hewitt, Sarah Passino, Sonalini Sapra, Ali Sevilla, Susan Saegert, Shubhra Sharma, and Anastasia Curwood. It was a gift to have so many great minds helping me along this path. I appreciate the time, thought, energy, and encouragement you have given me.

Thank you to the Templeton Foundation, to Keith Meador, and to all the folks at the Center for Spirituality, Theology and Health at Duke University Medical Center for providing me with the time and space to make this book a reality.

To my parents, thank you for always believing in me, supporting me, listening to me, and loving me. Thank you for giving me a passion for learning. You will forever be my first and favorite teachers, and my biggest cheerleaders. Finally, to Ryon and to Amy, thank you for supporting my dreams, for making me laugh, and for reminding me of what is important.

INTRODUCTION

CONSIDER TAM, A WOMAN who grew up in a home where her alcoholic stepfather, a well-regarded clinician, was emotionally abusive, yet revered.[1] Tam started drinking when she was eleven, and was addicted to alcohol and using other drugs by the time she reached high school. She suffered untreated mental illness during most of her childhood, and had been married and divorced three times by the time she was nineteen. Growing more ill and less financially independent with each divorce, Tam eventually ended up living on the streets of Nashville, Tennessee. Tam spent nearly thirty years on the streets, prostituting herself to the men who frequent Dickerson Road, and using the money she earned on drugs, alcohol, food, and when available, a place to sleep at night.

Three years ago, with a record of over ninety arrests and more than a dozen felony convictions, Tam entered Magdalene House, a recovery community that provides women with free housing, food, health care, dental care, psychological services, job training, and education, as well as gainful employment. The residential facility consists of four houses in which the women live, unsupervised, in the practice of healing community. The community's ethos is marked by paradoxical discourses: of healing that comes from brokenness, of security gained through vulnerability, and of independent selves made possible by commitments to others. The guiding belief of the community is evident in the bold but simple tagline added to all their materials: *Love heals.*

For Tam, and for more than a hundred other women who have entered the doors of Magdalene since its opening in 1997, healing is no small undertaking. Women come off the streets malnourished, ad-

1

dicted, isolated, and carrying the effects of years of suffering. Of the twenty-two women in residence at Magdalene at the time of this study, approximately 80 percent had been diagnosed with a mental illness other than addiction, 40 percent were receiving treatment for hepatitis C, and roughly one-third were HIV positive. Still, members of the Magdalene community are far more than sufferers or victims—women don't survive on the streets for years by being weak, unlucky, or stupid. They survive by being strong, savvy, and as many of them believe, "protected by God." When a woman enters Magdalene, the healing that begins to take place is a powerful process that requires an equally powerful community to help her strength of survival transform into health and flourishing. Magdalene's stories of healing instruct us that true health requires the redemption and renewal of mind, body, and spirit. Furthermore, healing relies on deep friendship that is long-standing, unconditional, and fostered in community. As Toni, a Magdalene graduate, describes it: "My relationships at Magdalene and Thistle Farms . . . make me believe that no matter what I have done or experienced, they still love me. Just hold on, hold on. It's gonna get better. I'm gonna get better."

When I write about Tam, Toni, and the other women I met while conducting ethnographic research in the Magdalene community, I feel as though I am describing characters from a movie or a novel—characters whose experiences mirror reality but ultimately seem like hyperbolic accounts constructed for the purpose of sensational storytelling. Unfortunately, Tam is not a fictional character, and her experiences are not exaggerated. In fact, they are quite typical for a growing number of people in the United States; such experiences seem sensational only because they are often hidden from sight. According to conservative estimates, each year in the United States almost 1 million children are abused or neglected (USD HHS 2007); 2.5 million adults struggle with substance abuse (SAMHSA 2009); 100,000 women participate in street-based sex work (*ProCon.org* 2008); and 1.6 million people experience homelessness (USD HUD 2009). The people represented by these statistics are frequently surrounded by system-based barriers that hold them hostage to such experiences: lack of access to appropriate treatment, affordable housing, and gainful employment can mean that abuse, addiction, and the like will be their lifelong companions. Currently, in the United States, all forms of prostitution are illegal in most states. They are considered criminal violations against the public order in every state except two: Rhode Island and Nevada. In Rhode Island, sex work that takes place indoors is legal, and in Nevada, sex work and brothels are permissible in counties with fewer than 400,000 residents. Additionally, there are many sex workers and escort agencies throughout the United States that work and advertise under the auspices of "body work" and "escorting" (Milio, Peltier, and Hufnail 2000). While this is not technically legal, it is largely ignored by authorities, and prostitution thus flourishes as a lucrative establishment in many major metropolitan areas. Statistics demonstrate that prostitution is pervasive in the United States: the results of a 2004 poll by TNS, a global market research company, indicated that 15 percent of men have paid for sex, and 30 percent of single men over thirty have paid for sex (Langer, Arnedt, and Sussman 2004).

In addition to examining what one might call the traditional moral issues surrounding the practice and legality of exchanging money for sex, feminist scholars and activists have engaged in discussing a somewhat different moral dilemma: whether prostitution represents yet another example (and, some would argue, a most egregious one at that) of the exploitation of women's bodies for male pleasure, or whether it is a resourceful response to market demands. On the one hand, activists indicate that women often enter sex work (especially street-based prostitution) as a response to environments and situations that have left them few other options. For example, women overwhelmingly report financial pressures as the reason they entered the sex trade (Chapkis 1997; Mulia 2002; Vanwesenbeeck 2001). In some communities, engagement in prostitution is viewed as the most desperate response to dire economic situations, and a symbol of the extent to which the community has deteriorated (Durr 2005). Other activists point to the high correlation between involvement in sex work and childhood abuse, and between involvement in sex work and substance abuse. From each of these perspectives, women trade their sexual services for money because of desperation or past exploitation.

Alternatively, other women assert that sex work is the most interesting and viable employment option available (Petro 2007), and though it may be far from ideal, it is preferable to other opportunities such as cleaning houses (Chua, Bhavani, and Foran 2000) or performing secretarial work (Chapkis 1997). Still others argue that although sex work is not a desirable occupation, it is the work available to them, and as such, the fact that they are working should be respected. While these women are more likely to acknowledge their involvement in sex work as economically coerced, they often object to the idea that they are without agency. For them, sex work is a site of resistance (Chua, Bhavani, and Foran 2000; Chapkis 1997; Kempadoo and Doezma 1998) and an active response to marginalizing economic structures and difficult life experiences.

Beyond these debates lie questions about whether or not prostitution is good for women. Although some argue that it is (or at least could be, given the proper set of legal protections and support), statistics demonstrate that street-based sex work is one of the most dangerous occupations in the world (Goodyear and Cusick 2007). In addition to the violence they experience on the streets, women involved in prostitution are far more likely than their male clients to incur punishment at the hands of legal authorities. Women participating in street-based sex work are the most subject to arrest (and to other forms of abuse as well). From 1994 to 2004, an estimated 73,800–100,200 prostitution arrests were made annually in the United States (*ProCon.org* 2008). Women who are arrested often suffer abuse from authorities such as police personnel and prison guards, and they are rarely given tools or resources for exiting prostitution should they so desire (Nagle 1997).

Some countries (such as England) have begun to acknowledge the lack of exit options; however, their ventures into providing programs to address this have proved to be challenging (O'Neill 2007). For example, according to needs assessment measures described by Margaret Melrose (2007), the most effective strategies for a holistic exit program require attention to health care, employment and housing needs, and sustainable funding. Such services are costly and difficult to deliver and coordinate.

Most of the women at Magdalene would say that drug addiction had provided the impetus for their involvement in sex work. The women I interviewed described a downward spiral in which they had used drugs recreationally, become addicted, needed to prostitute themselves in order to afford getting high, and needed to be high to perform the sex work. Although addiction is increasingly recognized as a complicated phenomenon that involves biological makeup, personal choice, social context, and family history (Brady and Back 2009), the women had often been denied treatment in favor of jail time or monetary fines, a practice that led them to continue using drugs and maintained their marginalization. The evidence suggests that this is a nationwide trend: between 1980 and 2004, the US prison population rose by 275 percent.[2] Seventy-four percent of this increase was linked to drug-related crimes, the majority of which were nonviolent. Furthermore, it appears that punishment for drug-related offenses is incurred more often by certain groups. Despite the fact that drug use is well distributed across factors such as race and social class, a disproportionate number of inmates are Latino or African American, and they are more likely to suffer from poverty, mental illness, addiction, or disabilities. Furthermore, "few correctional facilities mitigate the educational and/or skill deficiencies of their inmates, and most inmates will return home to communities that are ill equipped to house or rehabilitate them" (Golembeski and Fullilove 2005, 185). These deficiencies have serious effects on the persons released from prisons and the communities to which they return. Studies show that inmates leave poorer, sicker, and more marginalized than they were before incarceration (Biswanger et al. 2007; Golembeski and Fullilove 2005; Singer 2008). In addition to the human cost of such trends, the financial burdens are enormous: from 1990 to 2000, the federal government increased spending on correctional facilities by 521 percent, while cutting its spending on education and employment programs almost in half (Golembeski and Fullilove 2005).

Without a doubt, policies concerning prostitution and drug use influence women's experiences of them, as do the social meanings tied to these activities. They shape the ways in which women decline from recreational users to addicts on the street, and the ways in which they can and will seek treatment. On the other hand, it seems that these policies and social understandings have had little positive effect on prostitution and drug use. Furthermore, they fail to acknowledge addiction and sex work as complex experiences that vary from person to person. For example, some of the women I interviewed found prostitution empowering, at least in the beginning. Other women rebutted such claims, seeing prostitution as the last stop on an increasingly treacherous path that had been paved by drug use and a lifetime of physical and emotional pain. Still others were ambivalent about the practice. Similarly, women reported a variety of experiences with drug use and abuse, most of them beginning with drug use as an adventure, an antidote, or a way to numb pain. Regardless of the women's initial experiences with drug use and sex work, however, prostituting and getting high had eventually become an endless, all-encompassing cycle that they had all felt powerless to leave.

With this in mind, it seems that the best way to understand these experiences and the resources required to address them is to act "close to the ground"—to embark on research and develop strategies responsive to the needs and desires of individual women in particular contexts and communities. The purpose of this book is to tell the story of Magdalene as a community of healing—true healing—in a love-inspired journey toward wholeness. Furthermore, this book seeks a full definition of healing—one that goes beyond illness to talk about suffering, and expands the concept of suffering from an individual phenomenon to a social one.

In the opening chapters, I provide a description of the Magdalene community, and a survey of the many reasons women end up on the streets. During one of my first visits to Magdalene, I was talking with a staff member about social injustices of various sorts, particularly my concerns about how they arranged themselves along the lines of gender, race, class, and sexuality. As I rehearsed well-known sociological theories about the systemic reasons for the experiences that women at Magdalene had endured, she stopped me and said, "I think it's so important to talk about the things you're describing, but at the end of the day, you have to remember that those things all come together in the life of *one* person—that they're lived and experienced one unique person at a time." In the spirit of honoring the many "one persons" who have entered the doors of Magdalene, Chapter 3 offers the story of one woman, Marion, and her journey of illness and recovery.

In Chapter 4, I explore dimensions of healing as described and experienced by the women in the Magdalene community. A common expression I heard describes a person as "clean but not recovered." This phrase was used to illustrate that a person could be rid of an illness (in this case, addiction) that had been medically and socially ascribed to her without being truly well. Health and wellness for the women at Magdalene meant far more than the absence of illness. They required healing and growth of the total person—body, mind, and soul—as well as attention to the person's relationships with others and the world surrounding her.

Chapters 5 and 6 describe specific aspects of Magdalene that community members identified as essential to their processes of healing. Chapter 5 pays close attention to the spiritual commitments of the Magdalene community and the ways such commitments inform beliefs about the role of hospitality in the effort to support recovery. In Chapter 6, I relay community members' accounts of the love and acceptance they have experienced at Magdalene, and contrast this with their experiences of rejection and marginalization in other communities, recovery programs, and jails and prisons. According to Magdalene residents and staff, one of the unique aspects of the community is its commitment to providing ample time and space for recovery to occur. Community members often talk about the mystery and creativity involved in healing the self and others, asserting that these qualities can develop only in an environment that provides room for revisiting the past, closing old wounds, and dreaming of the future.

In an epistemological era in which making claims of "truth" put the speaker at risk for accusations of naïveté, oversimplification, or hegemony, women from Magdalene participate in an ongoing practice of speaking truth in love. The practice entails speaking at public events, publishing written material, and positing a vision of feminism and flourishing in which it is wrong to buy and sell women. Chapter 7 explores the truth claims made by women at Magdalene, the ways such truths are dispersed, and the complexities involved with spreading the message of Magdalene beyond the community from which it originates.

Despite Magdalene House's reputation of treatment success, barriers to healing often remain powerful obstacles for women in the community. Furthermore, these multiple barriers are rooted as much in social, political, and economic systems as they are in individual women, their immediate families, and their communities. It would be nice to believe that once healing occurs, they—and we—never go back to a place of isolation or illness. But the reality of life in general, and addiction specifically, is that the process of healing and recovery is a winding journey—one in which we often find ourselves right back in the very places we never thought we would again be.

CHAPTER 1

Magdalene

M Y FIRST EXPOSURE TO the Magdalene House program took place during my first year of graduate school. One of my professors assigned a project for which each student had to observe a local service organization and conduct an evaluation using a particular theoretical model. I waded through hundreds of websites for local nonprofit organizations, but none of the groups seemed as compelling as Thistle Farms, a small cooperative bath and body care company run by the women of Magdalene House. I imagined myself pursuing my research while surrounded by strong and purposeful women, immersed in a lovely world of lavender fragrance and handicrafts. I called the number for the Magdalene offices and was greeted by a rough voice that said:

"You mean you wanna be an intern?"

"No, not exactly. I'm doing a project for class, and—"

"We don't really do that." Click.

I ended up focusing on an adult literacy program for that assignment, and soon started working with professors in places far more glamorous than Nashville (at least in my mind). I spent one summer in Ecuador and another in Argentina. I traveled to Kenya and Alaska. I learned about research ethics and socialized medicine from Costa Rican physicians and scientists. Then, four years after my initial phone call, I heard that Magdalene needed an intern coordinator, and I jumped at the chance.

When I arrived at Magdalene's main house, at the corner of Booker and Lena Streets, the three women talking and laughing on the front

porch responded nicely to my hello, but without any apparent interest: it was clear that people came and went often, and my arrival was
hardly a reason to interrupt a smoke break. Inside, sitting on an over-
stuffed couch, was the woman I would come to know as Miss Minda,
one of Magdalene's most colorful residents. Miss Minda loved wigs; to
see her looking like Tina Turner one day and Goldilocks the next was
not uncommon. Two women rushed through the front door, introducing themselves as Becca, Magdalene's executive director, and Claire,
its director of public relations.

During our meeting, we hammered out my duties as intern coordinator, which I would perform as a volunteer, and devised a plan for me
to learn more about Magdalene in time to teach the incoming interns
about the organization. Our meeting was a little "loose," for lack of a
better term—we spent as much time off topic as on, and there was an
underlying expectation that I would figure things out as I went along.
The looseness of the meeting is somewhat illustrative of Magdalene
in general: there are rules, but they are not always hard-and-fast; there
is leadership, but not a lot of hand-holding; there is structure and tradition, but it is perpetually subject to creative reinterpretation. These
qualities, while sometimes frustrating, also seem to give Magdalene
some of its power and charm.

After the meeting, one of Magdalene's many volunteers stepped
out of an office to give me a tour. Cristen led me around the house,
pointing out different aspects of its construction ("It was designed by a
female architect who was familiar with the program") and offering various personal observations ("These baseboards clearly need dusting").
The house, officially named "The Anne Stevens Community House"
in honor of Becca's mother, is more often simply called "Lena." The
newest and largest of Magdalene's five residences at the time, it houses
eight women, each of whom has her own small bedroom, as well as the
organization's main administrative offices and a meeting room. There
is also ample common space: a kitchen with two stoves and two re-
frigerators, a living room with comfortable couches and a large-screen
television, and an outdoor prayer garden located just off the living
room. In the two years I volunteered and conducted research at Mag-

dalene, I never came to Lena when it wasn't bustling—it was always full of people, activity, and noise.

The Beginning

There are different versions of Magdalene's short history, and I've heard it told several ways. No one seems entirely sure where or how it started, but they all agree that it involved Becca Stevens, an unconventional and charismatic Episcopal priest who grew up in Nashville, married a songwriter, preaches barefoot, and traverses the traditional lines drawn by race, class, and creed with uncanny ease. As far as I've been able to determine, the idea for Magdalene came to Becca and a handful of others while they were visiting women in jails and prisons. During their visits, they noticed that although there were several transition programs for men leaving correctional facilities, there were few for women, and none for women with histories of addiction and involvement in sex work. Becca describes the beginning phase:

> When I first started the project, I said that I wanted to do what the women who would eventually be in the program would want to be done. So we started interviewing women in jail, because I couldn't figure out what the issues were or what we were doing. There wasn't a vision or a philosophy or a theology that was really well figured out. There were inklings, and there were dreams, and hopes. And that's when I started going down to jail and met people that I could have easily switched place with. People that I had graduated high school with and all that. So the philosophy, I guess, was that I wanted to set up something that way I would want it done for me.

As Becca and others began stumbling through implementing such a program, they had a few false starts. One was providing a handful of women coming out of prison with bunks and rooms at an already established residential transition community for men. It quickly became clear that this was, in Becca's words, "a really bad idea," and that the women needed a place of their own. In 1996, Magdalene became incorporated as its own organization and started renting a house on the ironically named Park Avenue in a rundown area of Nashville. Until August 1997, Becca raised money, continued to meet with women in jails and prisons, pastored her own church, and gathered people willing to help her further the Magdalene vision. In the second week of August in 1997, the newly renovated Park Avenue house opened its doors to five women whom the Tennessee women's prison had agreed to release on the condition that they participate in the Magdalene program. The women attended therapy groups and job-training classes at the YWCA, participated in twelve-step meetings, fought often enough to merit outside intervention, and went on retreats in the Smoky Mountains.[1] All five of the women stuck with the program for two years, stayed sober, and laid the groundwork for what it means to live in healing community. The pilot project proved successful enough to garner additional interest and financial support from others in Nashville, which allowed the program to grow. Describing how she became one of Magdalene's longest-serving and most active volunteers, Corina said:

> Well, I went to the very first fundraiser — it was at Becca's house, I think — and I thought the program was an amazing program. And at that point, I don't think any of us really understood how incredible it was. I don't think Becca, even with her vision, realized how it would grow and what it would become. And over the years, we've just learned as we've gone along. When I quit working, I made an appointment with Becca, and just went in and said, "Here I am. This is where the Lord wants me to be." And she said, "Well, what does the Lord want you to do?" And I said, "I haven't got a clue. Just use me wherever you can." So we would just find a thing here and a thing there.

The things here and things there that Corina has done at Magdalene include everything from sewing eye pillows to chairing the fundraiser, from wiping down candles to serving as president of the board of directors. In the way that Becca's original plan for Magdalene started as "inklings," the program in 1997 was a small but convincing glimpse of what it would eventually become. In 1998, it opened another house on Hillside Drive, and in 1999 it opened a third building on Arthur Avenue. In 2000, someone gave the program the plot of land at the corner of Lena and Booker Streets, and the community conducted a capital campaign to build what is now its main house. In 2001, it started Thistle Farms. By the time Magdalene celebrated its tenth anniversary, in 2007, it owned five residences and a small but growing cooperative business. It employed nine staff members, including Sonya, the program director, whom the residents frequently described as "a woman of purpose." Most importantly, over a hundred women had completed the Magdalene program, and the majority of them remain sober, employed, housed, and out of prison. What makes Magdalene successful is something of a mystery, although its staff, volunteers, residents, and graduates agree that some of the most important ingredients are a community marked by love and acceptance, full and free provision of multiple services, and the time and space to grow and heal.

The Program

The underlying principle of "Do unto others . . ." runs consistently throughout Magdalene programming, as do themes of love and acceptance. "Love," however, is more than emotion, and the Golden Rule is more than principle. They are conveyed through the provision of resources deemed basic and necessary for all human beings, including (and especially) women living in prison or on the streets. For example, during the time that women live at Magdalene, they receive medical and dental treatment, psychological counseling, education, and job skills training, all at no cost to them. Additionally, each woman receives a stipend during her first three months at Magdalene; she is free to use the money as she determines, except to buy alcohol or illicit drugs. The narrative that surrounds Magdalene names it as a recovery community unlike any other (or at least unlike any other that the women have ever experienced). When asked, "What sets Magdalene apart?," its staff and residents are quick to agree: the length of time (two years) it allows for recovery, its comprehensive and holistic approach to healing, and the expectation that its residents will live in community and be treated with dignity.

THE HOUSES

When a woman enters the Magdalene program, she is immediately given a key to the house in which she will live, assigned to a bedroom in that house, and informed that she will have unlimited access to all the other amenities in the house. While there are staff members who check on the houses to ensure that repairs are performed, there are no staff members who serve as authorities in the houses themselves. The philosophy of Magdalene trusts the community created by the women living together to serve as the authority. Explaining the reasoning behind this, Becca said:

> I think it's really different to have no staff living in the houses at all. So everybody that lives in the houses that are opened at Magdalene are part of the community, and they have ownership of it. I have never had a key to any of Magdalene's homes. Never. I've always had to ask to come in. When someone comes to my house, they're my guest. And I wanted to set it up so that I could be—had to be—a guest in the house of the women.

I quickly learned that the simple beauty of the houses and the opportunity for "ownership" were as important to the women who live at Magdalene as they were for Becca. Kathleen told me about seeing the house on Lena Street for the first time:

> I can remember when Marion and them took me to the house on Lena, and here was this beautiful house, and I was like, "This is the house I *prayed for* when I was in my addiction," and to know what I came from, and where I'd been and to see that blessing, just that *house*—I kissed the floor. Because dreams just don't—prayers don't come true like that. Not from where I come from—you can pray for another hit, but you can't pray for a way out. And to get it? Oh my God! And, a key? My own key? To a house that was like a mansion?

Many other women described similar feelings of astonishment when they left the streets or prison and came to Lena. They talked about the thrill of being in a place that was beautiful, safe, and clean, and described the house as "a light," "a sanctuary," and "a blessing." The other Magdalene houses are somewhat less spectacular, but nonetheless places of safety and comfort. Becca talked at length about the importance of the houses:

> Where other people may have put some really good program pieces in place, I made welcome baskets and put nice sheets on the Sealy Posturepedic beds. We actually had a specific donor for good beds, because I kept thinking I really wanted it to be so comfortable. If you've been on those jail cots when you go in the prisons—they're just so hard. And you go on the streets and women are literally sleeping under bridges and stuff, and I just thought, "You know, if that were me, I'd want a really sweet little lamp, and a good bed, and I'd want everybody to leave me the hell alone, and I wouldn't want anybody bossing me around."

Each year, groups from outside Nashville visit Magdalene in hopes of learning enough to replicate at least some aspects of the program in their own communities. During these visits, Magdalene invites the guests to tour the residences and Thistle Farms, sit in on meetings, view the annual budgets, and ask any question they can come up with. The idea that all the women live in the houses without supervision inevitably provokes the strongest reactions. Some visitors are inspired by the idea and others are repelled, but they all ask the same questions: Does it work? Can you really bring women in off the streets and trust them to live unsupervised?

Julie, a woman who runs a program called "Bloom!" in collaboration with a drug and prostitution court in Columbus, Ohio, talked with me briefly about bringing members of her program and the drug court with her to visit Magdalene. A member of her group repeatedly asked Magdalene staff and residents about the keys the residents receive when they first arrive. She was in such disbelief that the women could be their own authority to come and go responsibly that she could not seem to get her mind around the idea. As the day went on, however, one by one, the members of Julie's group went from being skeptics to believing in the way Magdalene conducts business. "We finally got it," Julie said. "If you treat women like prisoners, they'll act like prisoners. If you treat women like women, they'll act like women."

The commitment to dignity and equality is evident throughout Magdalene community practices, as is a profound commitment to mercy. Mercy is demonstrated in countless ways, but perhaps it begins with offering women the opportunity to come off the streets to comfortable houses in which to rest and heal.

THE PROCESS OF HEALING

During the first week or two that a woman lives at Magdalene, she does little more than rest. Particularly for women who come directly from the streets, this time is essential for reestablishing habits as basic as eating and sleeping. Describing her process at Magdalene, Kayla said, "It took me two months to relearn how to go to bed at night and get up in the morning. I was so used to being up for days at a time—never sleeping, never eating, never bathing." In addition to resting, women typically undergo mental and physical health assessments, and many of them see a dentist for the first time in years.

During the second or third week, the woman begins a ninety-day intensive outpatient (IOP) treatment. Magdalene contracts with Centerstone, a large mental health provider in the state of Tennessee, to provide the IOP services, and the women travel to Centerstone daily to attend twelve-step meetings, counseling sessions, and other treatment activities. During the first ninety days, Magdalene also provides each woman with a small weekly stipend so that she can buy food or cigarettes without having to worry about where the money is going to come from. According to Becca, this is one of the most generous things that Magdalene does for the women:

> It's always hard when you're struggling with no money, and I know the women coming out of jail don't have any money, and so I just wanted to erase that. I didn't want women to have to go back to the men they

were tricking on the streets just to buy a pack of cigarettes or groceries or nail polish. So that's where we came up with the idea of "We're going to pay you to stay for the first ninety days. You're not going to pay us; we're going to pay you."

Becca contrasted Magdalene with other programs and halfway houses where residents have to pay for housing, food, and other necessities. While this model is relatively common, staff and residents at Magdalene say that requiring someone to pay $125 a week to live in recovery housing ignores the realities of coming out of jail or off the streets. For women who have little or no work history, this type of requirement only leads them back to the streets, since the quickest and most accessible way to make money is through prostitution or selling drugs. Furthermore, the idea of running a recovery program for financial profit seems unthinkable to many members of the community. Marion, a Magdalene graduate and staff member, related this practice to another that she clearly sees as exploitative when she said, "I mean, are [the for-profit centers] promoting recovery or pimping people? *Seriously*."

Ironically, the provision of a stipend is often one of the first things that forces a woman at Magdalene to rely on her community. Although many women manage to save and spend the money on their own within the confines of the community's rules for its use, others have to ask their "Magdalene sisters" to help them resist the temptation to spend it on drugs. Lacy, one of the early Magdalene graduates, credits Nancy, another graduate, for "saving me from my stipend" (a phrase she always said with a laugh). Each week, after receiving the money, Lacy would give it to Nancy and say, "I can't handle this. I need you to hold this, and only give it to me when I ask you to and need something specific. Don't ever give me more than five dollars at a time." Her friend was faithful: Lacy eventually got to the point where she could handle her stipend and no longer needed Nancy to hold it for her. The lesson she learned, however—how to ask for help, and how to trust people to give it to her—is a tool she continues to use in her recovery many years later.

After the ninety-day IOP phase is over, the women spend the next eight to twelve weeks enrolled in computer training at an adult education facility that provides free services to residents of Davidson County. Jeff, a member of the Magdalene program staff, explained that the role of the computer training is twofold: it teaches basic computer skills, and it gives the women time to ease into the responsibility of showing up consistently and on time to perform a work-related task. Throughout the IOP treatment and computer training, the staff of Magdalene works with each new resident to develop an individual plan for obtaining necessary physical and mental health services and achieving long-term goals. Additionally, the staff works with the woman to address any unfulfilled responsibilities such as outstanding warrants, unpaid child support, or other debt. They allow and encourage each woman to identify her own interests when it comes to education and vocational training, but require her to work toward her GED if she does not already have a GED or high school diploma.

After completing IOP treatment and computer training, most women seek employment at Thistle Farms. Thistle Farms was started when staff and residents at Magdalene discovered how difficult it was for the residents to find legal employment. There is a range of employment experiences and capacities among the women; however, many of them have criminal records, and some have never held a legal job. At Thistle Farms, the women create high-quality bath and body products that are "as kind to the environment as they are to the body" (Thistle Farms 2008). Rituals of healing and wholeness run throughout the practices of Thistle Farms: each workday begins with a meditation (also known as "the circle"), the products are sold at events where women tell their stories, and all proceeds go back into the community of Magdalene. Thistle Farms is open from 9:00 a.m. to 2:00 p.m. three days a week and employs about twenty Magdalene residents and graduates. The women are encouraged to spend their paychecks as they wish. However, Magdalene offers each woman an individual investment account and matches each dollar saved to the account. The woman is able to withdraw the money when she leaves, to spend on school, a car, or housing.

Like the rest of Magdalene, Thistle Farms began small and pro-
gressed creatively, driven by a combination of need and inspiration.
Holli Anglin, the longtime director of Thistle Farms, described what
the company was like when she first began working there:

> February 14, 2001, was the official launch of Thistle Farms, and
> I started volunteering the following summer, and then was hired
> that fall. When I started out, it was truly "organic," shall we say. For
> example, there were no books, really—no bookkeeping. I walked in
> and a staff member grabs me by the hand and says, "Here's all the
> accounting, here's some folders, here's a box of some stuff that you
> might want . . . and here's a lunch table." And I thought, "Where are
> the computers? How does everything work?" I'm used to coming from
> a business environment where systems are already kind of in place.
> And when I got to Thistle Farms, there were no systems per se. So
> we were completely trying to figure it out together. It was pretty—it
> was exciting, but it was intimidating. And it was definitely true in the
> sense of a start-up company. We were at St. Augustine's Chapel and
> we would set up these lunch tables every day. . . . We made just a few
> products: a candle, a body balm, a lip gloss—that might have been
> it. Thistle Farms employed me and six Magdalene residents. Now we
> employ twenty women, have far more products and scents, and have a
> much bigger facility. We've improved from a quality standpoint too, I
> think. But the basics are still the same.

On the days that the residents are not working, there are a number
of activities available to them, including spirituality groups, art classes,
writing classes, and community meetings. As women near the end of
their time at Magdalene, the program offers them several options, including continuation of their employment at Thistle Farms (if they are
working there already), space in a one-year transitional home, or support in finding an apartment or home of their own. The recommended
period of residency at Magdalene is two years; however, some women
leave early, either because they are ready to move on or because they
have relapsed. For women who stay in the community for at least thirty

days, the recovery rate is over 70 percent, which is far higher than that of most recovery programs (Gossop, Stewart, and Marsden 2007; Hubbard et al. 1998).

Magdalene's retention rate and success (measured by sobriety, employment, and stable residence) is especially impressive considering the population it serves. In the general population, treatment completion is more likely for clients who abuse alcohol as their primary substance, have at least a high school education, are thirty years old or older upon entering treatment, have stable employment, and are non-Hispanic white males (SAMHSA 2009). Conversely, crack cocaine and heroin are the typical drugs of choice for Magdalene residents; most lack employment, most did not complete high school, and all are female. According to the residents and graduates for whom Magdalene was successful, there are many important differences between Magdalene and other treatment programs. Women mentioned the long-term nature of the program as an aspect that allowed them time to heal spiritually and psychologically as well as physically. They emphasized that recovery was about more than just being clean, and that true recovery takes time and multiple forms of support, including that of a loving community.

THE SUPPORT OF HEALING

The opportunities and structures that support healing and recovery require a tremendous amount of resources, both monetary and otherwise. The community of Magdalene is maintained by a large network of staff, donors, and volunteers. Magdalene and Thistle Farms have a combined staff of ten, including an executive director, a Magdalene program director, four Magdalene program staff (two of whom are licensed counselors, and two of whom are Magdalene graduates), an education coordinator, a Thistle Farms director, and two public relations and development staff. The staff is mixed in terms of age and race; however, they are all women, with the exception of one man on the program staff.

In addition, the community is supported by several different agencies (for example, Interfaith Dental provides dental care and Siloam Health Clinic provides medical care), as well as hundreds of dedicated volunteers who do everything from planning the annual fundraiser to repairing the residences. The volunteers represent a range of ages and include both men and women. For the most part, they have disposable resources in terms of either money or time. The volunteer newsletter is e-mailed to over a thousand individuals in the Nashville area. Although most of these volunteers donate time or money to Magdalene once or twice a year, some of them spend countless hours each week contributing to the Magdalene community. For example, Ruth, a retired teacher, schedules every sales event and many speaking engagements for Thistle Farms. Her work includes identifying potential hosts and contacting them, managing the logistics of the events (including time, space, location, directions, speakers, and inventory), and writing thank you notes. Sales and speaking events generally occur once or twice a week; however, the holiday season of 2008 was busy enough to include between ten and twelve events each week. Ruth's efforts are essential to the success of Thistle Farms, and her work for the company is full time. Although nearly all the volunteers at Magdalene or Thistle Farms are there because they want to help, most of them would also say that they volunteer because it contributes to their own well-being. As one volunteer often says to the residents working at Thistle Farms, "I don't know if you need to be here, but I know *I* do."

Although no one I interviewed said this directly, my observations led me to conclude that another key difference between Magdalene and other recovery programs was that most of the staff and volunteers at Magdalene do not have a background in psychology or social work. Their vocations range from priest to accountant to massage therapist, and their connections to the community are just as varied. Without a doubt, the therapy and treatment the women receive at Magdalene are *essential* to their recovery. However, the presence of individuals besides mental health professionals and caseworkers creates an environment in which the residents and graduates are seen primarily as *people*, not as clients. Additionally, for many of the staff and volunteers, the women's stories are not far from their own: among the staff and volunteers I interviewed, several had personal or family experiences of addiction and abuse. Although Magdalene stands firmly against prostitution as a legal or legitimate practice, many of the women, staff, and volunteers

join feminist critics in saying that the exchange of sex for money (or resources or power or myriad other things) is not a practice restricted to
dark streets and back alleys. Although they are aware of the systems of
racism, sexism, and poverty that have affected the lives of the women
who come to Magdalene, the community's residents, graduates, staff,
and volunteers are quick to make connections that reach across traditional analyses and demonstrate the similarities between people and
experiences as well as the differences. Talking about the popularity of
the program with donors and volunteers, Becca reflected on why she
thought people felt so connected to the issues of addiction and prostitution: "There is a mystique about it and I think everybody knows there's
a part of themselves that's a part of it, too—that we sell ourselves to
get something else." This explanation falls in line with something else
I have heard Becca say on many occasions: "The line between priest
and prostitute is very small."

Magdalene's budget for fiscal year 2008–2009 was approximately
$557,000, which covered all Magdalene and Thistle Farms expenses.
These included repairs, maintenance, supplies, and utilities for the
houses; medical, dental, and mental health care for residents; staff
wages; and other program needs. Magdalene's cost per day for each of
its twenty-two residents was $44.00; this figure included all occupancy,
transportation, and payroll expenses, as well as the costs associated with
treatment, educational, and vocational services. By contrast, the per
diem rate at prison facilities for women in Tennessee was $87.98.

In its first eleven years of existence, Magdalene was able to raise
enough money to meet or exceed its budget each year, and did so
largely through individual donations. Individuals donated approximately $360,000 during 2007–2008, and private organizations or con-
gregations contributed another $150,000. The remainder of the money
was generated through grants (mostly from local foundations), and
income from the Prostitution Solicitation School, which Magdalene
runs in collaboration with Nashville's police department, district attorney's office, and public defender's office.[2] Magdalene does not receive
any direct government funding; rather, it relies on the money and time
given by its donors and volunteers.

The presence of such a large network and the commitment of its members indicate the tremendous amount of resources required to assist women coming off the streets, as well as the importance of the work. Furthermore, for many involved, the provision of resources for women who have been without is not an act of charity—it is a restoration of justice. One volunteer told me, "The women shouldn't feel shame. The shame lies with society. Society has . . . I don't want to say 'betrayed them,' but . . . society hasn't supported them in the way in which they deserve to be supported."

The Spiritual Roots of the Community

In addition to the programmatic pieces that define Magdalene House, a deep spirituality informs its work and practice as a healing community. There are several scholars in the fields of psychology and psychiatry who believe that addressing spirituality is essential for patients for whom it is important (Pargament 2007). At Magdalene, however, spirituality is deemed important for all who are seeking the path to recovery and healing. Moreover, the values and worldview expressed by faithfulness to a God concerned about a suffering but beautiful world supply the narrative through which the community has formed its identity and performs its work.

Unlike many organizations that have grown from particular faith traditions, Magdalene is difficult to pin down as "faith-based." In many ways, Magdalene is profoundly rooted in beliefs about love, mercy, and the sacredness of life. Attention to Christian teachings and devotion to God provide meaning and purpose to many in the community. Benedictine theology guides the way in which the residences were designed and the workday at Thistle Farms is ordered. Prayer has a central place in the daily practices of Magdalene. Still, many of the staff, volunteers, and residents shy away from the idea that Magdalene is a religious place—or, at least the type of place they generally associate with the word "religious." Rather, the women of Magdalene have developed something of a grassroots theology—one that has at its center a God who suffers and a God who heals.

In 2008, the women of Magdalene published a book called *Find*

Your Way Home: Words from the Street, Wisdom from the Heart, in which different voices from the community articulate the meanings behind twenty-four principles that are set out in the book as the Rule of Magdalene. Each principle represents a guideline for living developed from beliefs about God that were worked out through the experiences and practices of community. Among the principles are admonitions such as "Proclaim original grace," "Find your place in the circle," "Think of the stranger as God," "Stand on new ground and believe you are not lost," "Show hospitality to all," "Love without judgment," and "Live in gratitude." Becca writes that the purpose of the book "is to share our truth that in community, love and grace are the most powerful forces of individual and social change. . . . [These] are stories of hope reminding us all that in whatever brokenness we know, the seeds of healing are sown" (Stevens 2008, 10–11). These beliefs are the starting point and the ending place of all of Magdalene's work, says Becca, and straying from them would have dire consequences for the community. The beliefs ground the work of Magdalene in a commitment to love, a trust in provision, and a responsibility to participate in the work of helping others to flourish.

Research Concerns, Process, and Limitations

My participation in the work of Magdalene started shortly after my initial meeting at Lena House. In 2007, I coordinated four student interns who were spending the summer in Nashville to fulfill one type of educational requirement or another. My work included meeting with them, learning about their interests, and introducing them to people within the organization with whom they fit. It also included helping them develop projects to meet internship requirements, and monitoring the progress of their projects. One of my goals was to help them see broader connections between the women they encountered at Magdalene and larger social, economic, and cultural phenomena. Unsurprisingly to anyone who has done work of this sort, my efforts to expand their perspectives led me to become more reflective about my own role in the community. At the end of the summer, I approached members of the community about conducting ethnographic research at Magdalene. The response was overwhelmingly positive and welcoming (something that I came to know as typical of the community), so I began the process of determining the most epistemologically and ethically appropriate way to capture the story of Magdalene.

Over the next two years, and throughout my research, I continued to volunteer at Magdalene as the intern coordinator. I also became a regular volunteer at Thistle Farms. I spent time there each Monday and Wednesday, and undertook tasks ranging from communicating with customers to grant writing to helping women complete their paperwork for food stamps. During this time, I came to consider myself a member of the community, and therefore approached my research as something of an insider. I believe that the lens of inquiry allowed me some critical distance; however, I do not believe that this research — or any other research, for that matter (Denzin and Lincoln 2005; Gebhardt 1982) — is purely objective. I believe that my deep involvement with the community was my greatest methodological tool, but also a methodological limitation.

As I began to explore the nature of the Magdalene community and the stories of its members, I was painfully aware of the many types and experiences of exploitation created by research itself, and of well-known abuses of research. In particular, feminist and postcolonial scholars have demonstrated the dangers of representation (or misrepresentation) in the knowledge creation process, even by scholars who are well meaning and attentive to issues of place and power (Foster-Fishman et al. 2003; Parpart 2002). For these theorists, research participants or subjects of study who have been marginalized because of various sociocultural phenomena (such as colonization or race and class hierarchies) are especially vulnerable to misrepresentation in scholarly pursuits. Indeed, some argue that accurate representation and understanding of marginalized groups is impossible (Spivak 1988); others argue that while it is possible, it requires a great deal of care, reflection, and accountability (Alcoff 1991).

The research on women involved in sex work provides a more specific demonstration of the implications for research and representation. For example, according to pro–sex work activists, street prostitution is over-studied precisely because it fulfills our expectations of "prostitution." In other words, these activists say that when people think of women involved in prostitution, they want to believe that all such women experience the horrors of the streets, as opposed to believing that there are women who exchange sex for money in safe, comfortable environments, and do so out of choice rather than desperation. While the argument that street prostitution is over-studied is contested, as is that of street prostitution as the prevailing image of women involved in sex work, there is growing consensus that the research on women involved in street prostitution has worked to cast them as images rather than as humans (Vanwesenbeeck 2001).

Nina Mulia (2000) describes how research and programmatic emphasis on disease concerns (particularly the HIV status) of drug-abusing women involved in prostitution has resulted in essentializing these individuals as disease vectors and dangerous women. These misrepresentations are important for practical as well as ideological reasons: they influence the type of care (or punishment) the women incur, perpetuate deep-seated beliefs about the appropriate bounds of female sexuality, and stand as justification for regulating it (Ringdal 1997). Beliefs about prostitutes as carriers of disease are not new, nor is the practice of developing regulatory guidelines based on gendered notions of sexuality and disease. History tells us that the concerns voiced by Mulia and others are not unfounded: in Great Britain during the 1800s, it was believed that only women could carry or transmit venereal diseases. As a result, women involved in prostitution could be picked up by law enforcement officials, forced to undergo medical examination, and institutionalized if they were diagnosed as infected. No such process existed for men who visited prostitutes (Pateman 1988; Ringdal 1997). While we now know that venereal disease can be and is carried and transmitted by men as well as women, the mechanisms for preventing and controlling it continue to assign different expectations and responsibilities to each gender in terms of sexual practices (Pateman 1988).

My concerns about representation were exacerbated by other questions of ethics and methodology that have followed me throughout my research career: Is research important? Is it valuable to anyone other than the researcher whose career it is supporting? And if it is important and valuable, how is it practiced in a liberatory fashion? These are, of course, mostly questions of voice and power, and I am not the first to ask them. Methodologists from a number of different traditions — among them feminist research, postcolonial studies, critical theory, and participatory research — have asked these questions and come up with quite different answers. As I carefully approached the subject of conducting research at Magdalene, I sought the work of these scholars as guides, but also took solace in the realization that the women with whom I would be working were powerful — powerful in their abilities to decide what they did and did not want, powerful in their abilities to speak out when they did not agree, and powerful in their abilities to represent themselves and tell their own stories. Marsha Henry (2007) alerts us to this dynamic in her article on authenticity in the research process: she warns against assuming the "power of the researcher" as a given, and calls for an approach to research that recognizes the systems of relationships of power in any fieldwork situation as multiple and complex.

Because of these reasons, I pursued a collaborative approach to my research, asking participants to shape research questions, participate in analysis, and provide feedback on my work. I sought a knowledge production process that was democratic and participatory, though perhaps somewhat different than one I would have derived from classic participatory research paradigms. In his article on citizenship and democracy, Harry Boyte (2003) invokes John Dewey when he proposes a view of knowledge production "as a democratic power resource that suggest(s) a democracy of abundance, not of scarcity, different than zero-sum distributive power or the competitive, consumer culture" (3). This view assumes knowledge creation processes that rely on an epistemological commitment to the social nature of knowledge and the value of people's experiences as they engage with the world around them. According to this view, all people are the experts of their own lives and experiences. They are therefore entitled to participation in the production of knowledge and essential to its process.

For the purposes of this project, collaboration in research took on two somewhat different forms. First, I had several formal and informal conversations with members of the community about their perspectives on the nature of the community, questions that they would like answered, and whom they thought I should ask for those answers. I allowed these conversations to guide me in the direction of the theories I used to form the framework of my study, and to guide the questions I asked in my qualitative interviews and focus groups. Second, I was aware of the strong value system of the community and chose to honor the norms and the struggles of importance to those within the community (Nagar 2002). I sought to turn the ethical commitments that informed the way that community was practiced into epistemological tools to uncover collective knowledge about the community itself. I set out to develop a methodology that recognized, drew on, and embraced the strengths and commitments of the women who make up the Magdalene community. I was able to ascertain these commitments during a year's worth of participation, observation, and conversations before my formal research project began. Through these activities, I came to the conclusion that my research must be, for ethical and epistemological reasons, based in shared experiences, reliant on storytelling, and grounded in relationship.

Most importantly, I learned about the community of Magdalene by participating in it. While I was conducting my research, the director of Thistle Farms said to me, "You know, people come to Thistle Farms all the time to do research, write newspaper stories—you know, to try to 'get us.' But it's just so hard—it's hard to understand, it's hard to know what's important. It's hard to know what questions to even ask. I like it that you've been here because you're one of us. You understand how things work and what needs to be done." In addition to feeling somewhat relieved that she had not seen my presence as a researcher as a burden, I felt affirmed in my belief that I could not have understood Magdalene and all that it does if I had spent only three months or six months or even a year there. The luxury of research support meant I had the opportunity to spend the time I needed with the community— nearly two years—to "get it." I was there when women came into the program, when they graduated, and when they relapsed. I was there for the deaths of family members, the births of grandchildren, and the excitement of adoptions. I saw people struggle and I saw them succeed.

I myself learned, grew, doubted, and hoped. In addition to witnessing and experiencing milestones, I also regularly engaged in the activities at Thistle Farms, which are in and of themselves creative pursuits. Residents, graduates, staff members, and volunteers often sit together to make bath and body products that will later be sold in a store or at a home party. The act of being in the same place and working on the same project is a partnership of sorts—a bonding experience. Because much of knowledge is created in the actions and silences of everyday living, being at Magdalene for more than just discourse was essential to my data collection.

The principles of action research alert us to the fact that in addition to the moral learning that occurs by participating in the process of social change, action is the best (and, some might argue, only) path to knowledge creation (Fals-Borda 1991; Kemmis and McTaggart 2000). In general, with action research, the type of action being spoken of is working for direct social change through political action or activism (Fals-Borda 1987, 1991). In many ways my presence at Thistle Farms would probably not be considered "activism"; however, I believe that my work alongside the women was an act of social change. I believe that without the action—the working alongside, the doing the stuff of life together—I could not have known the ins and outs of life in recovery as I do today. It was essential for me to be more than just an observer. It was essential for me to pour candles and to attend sales events. It was essential for me to give rides and to ask favors and to have enough in common that I shared *experiences*—not just conversations—with the people in my study.

To capture the day-to-day events of the Magdalene community, as well as the collective nature of the dialogues and relationships within it, I built on my shared experiences and conducted formal participant observation ten to fifteen hours a week over the course of three months. At the time, the community of Magdalene included four recovery houses, a transition home, and Thistle Farms, but I conducted participant observation only at Thistle Farms and at public Magdalene events such as book readings, resident graduation ceremonies, and community meetings. One of the tenets of Magdalene is that women should have the dignity of feeling at home and in control of their own homes. Because of this, and because Thistle Farms is the location of a large majority of community interactions, I conducted my participant observation at the company and purposely avoided doing so in the residences.

In addition to participant observation, I also conducted twenty-nine semi-structured qualitative interviews with current and former residents, graduates, staff, and volunteers. For the purposes of definition, "residents" are women who were living in one of the Magdalene houses at the time, "former residents" are women who had been a part of the community but left, "graduates" are women who lived in the community for approximately two years and completed program requirements, "staff" are people paid to work for Magdalene, and "volunteers" are people who work for Magdalene without monetary compensation. Making these distinctions is somewhat difficult, however, because people move from one category to another fairly often, and many occupy more than one category. For example, two members of the staff are graduates, volunteers often become staff, and the executive director is technically a volunteer in the sense that she is not paid, but she still occupies a place of centrality and authority. Nevertheless, I interviewed approximately 75 percent of the residents and staff. The number of volunteers I interviewed correspond to a much smaller proportion of the total number of volunteers who support Magdalene in any way; however, it is representative of the volunteers who provide substantial time and support to Magdalene. Finally, I conducted two group interviews, each of which involved approximately ten women either living at Magdalene or working at Thistle Farms or both. In these interviews, I engaged in an iterative process of discussing my findings with women in the community and incorporating their feedback into my analysis.

At the beginning of each workday at Thistle Farms, the person in charge of reading the meditation would say, "Let's open this meditation with a moment of silence followed by the Serenity Prayer." The Serenity Prayer, of course, is the mantra for virtually all twelve-step programs; the version recited at Thistle Farms is "God, grant me the serenity to accept the things I cannot change, the courage to change the

things I can, and the wisdom to know the difference, just for today."
The moment of silence is never very long, and I suppose it exists so
that everyone stops moving long enough to pay attention. It is a focusing exercise of sorts; at least it was for me. It isn't long enough to be a
time for prayer. At the end of the meditation, however, as we would
all stand with our arms around each other, the person who closes the
meditation would say, "Let's take a moment of silence for the sick and
suffering addict inside and out." This moment of silence is longer and
more purposeful, and as it takes place, I believe that people do think
about friends and family members who are still on the streets.

As I conducted my research, the second moment of silence reminded me to leave room in my analysis for the people who weren't
represented; to let their absence be known and to make space for their
claims and their concerns; and to acknowledge what might have been
said if their voices had been included in my project. With that in
mind, it is worth mentioning the limitations of this project. It would
have been advantageous to interview more women who had entered
the program but did not complete it. The two women I was able to
interview who fit this description still held very positive views of Magdalene, though there are likely women out there who do not. It would
have been interesting to know why these women chose not to stay at
Magdalene, and what it was about the community that failed to work
for them.

Additionally, there are at least a handful of other communities
in the United States that have modeled themselves after Magdalene
House in Nashville. I was able to interview the directors of two of these
programs; however, I do not provide extensive information about them.
Magdalene does not have a formal relationship with any of the organizations inspired by it, and the particularities of the programs are often
very different, although many of their commitments are the same. Exploring these other communities would provide an interesting look at
the commonalities and differences of the processes of healing that take
place in and through organizations such as Magdalene.

CHAPTER 2

The Path of Illness

How Women Get to Magdalene

I didn't wake up one day and decide, "I want to be a
junkie. I want to be a prostitute." There were things that
led me to that.

— Kayla, Magdalene House graduate

THERE IS NO FORMULA that neatly predicts a woman's progression to the streets. If you were to ask the women at Magdalene, "How did you get to Magdalene?" you would quickly realize that there is no one experience they all hold in common: many had abusive parents, but some had supportive parents; some grew up with drugs in their homes, others sought them out after they were living on their own; some lived on the streets for a matter of months, others for decades. When women explain the things that led them to life on the streets, they describe journeys that started many years ago and followed winding paths through unique places of strength and difficulty. At the same time, women often describe common themes of early abuse, frequent exposure to drugs and alcohol, and poor experiences with systems of authority. They talk about the comfort and the excitement they found in drugs and sex. And they talk about how difficult it was to find a place to heal once they had been battered by the streets and wanted a way out.

Early Experiences

Few of the women I interviewed described early childhood experiences that would be considered supportive of healthy human development. Twelve of the nineteen residents and graduates I interviewed described growing up in households marked by poverty and lack of access to appropriate, life-sustaining resources and services, and far more of them described chaotic and often harmful relationships. Because families are typically the primary context for child and adolescent development, economic or relational stress in those families has direct implications for human development (Caughy and O'Campo 2006; Kasper et al. 2008). In a society that does little to support alternative family configurations, stress is all but inevitable for families that do not fit the two-parent, dual wage-earner model. Importantly, this model was not typical for the women I interviewed: ten of the women had been raised by a single parent or caregiver, one by siblings, and two by foster parents. Although this wide variation is something that we would expect, former and current economic practices (such as the lack of a living wage) and sociocultural beliefs (such as identifying a two-heterosexual-parent household as the ideal for healthy childrearing) work to create environments in which some families thrive while others are denied basic necessities. For example, according to the US Census Bureau (2008), 1,759,000 single-parent families with children under eighteen had household earnings of $10,000 or less in 2008. For a family consisting of only a single parent and one child (which is seldom the case—for example, in my sample, women reported having between one and twelve siblings), this translates to approximately $13.70 per person per day to cover rent, utilities, food, clothing, health care, education, and all other expenses. This level of poverty often results in lack of adequate provision for the child (DeVoe et al. 2008), and it means that parents and caregivers are likely not receiving the services and support they need for themselves (Herman-Stahl et al. 2007; Lazear et al. 2008). Many of the women I interviewed talked about parents or caregivers who had unmet physical and mental health needs, and they were quick to link this to difficult or unstable home environments.

For the purposes of understanding the lives of women who end up at Magdalene, as well as general social practice and policy, it is important that pathology not be linked to individuals, families, or communities experiencing poverty as an inherent quality of those individuals, families, or communities. Nor do I mean to suggest belief in a culture of poverty, or to imply that experiences of mental illness, addiction, or abuse are constrained to families who fall below the poverty line. Rather, I mean to demonstrate that social ideologies and practices contribute to the existence and experience of poverty (Sen 1999; Nussbaum 2000), and that lack of resources can alter and exacerbate the consequences of addiction, abuse, and mental illness (Singer 2008), as we shall see.

ABUSE

Abuse and early childhood trauma (such as loss of a parent) were common themes in the stories the women told about their families and home lives. Fifteen women reported addiction in the home, and fourteen reported being physically or sexually abused at an early age (six by a parent or stepparent, one by a sibling, and seven by extended family members or close family friends).[1] Additionally, eight women described situations in which a parent or caregiver knew about the abuse that was occurring, but did not intervene. Four women reported having a parent or caregiver die while they were still children.

When Lisa told me her story, we were in the Magdalene program director's office. She sat in a chair by the window, and I sat with my back to the closed office door. As she talked about her childhood, slowly and unemotionally, she stared off into the space behind my head as if she could see the events of her childhood being replayed before her. She narrated a scene that was particularly salient in her memory:

> My mom got with another guy. And he was abusive. And he tried to rape me. My mom gave me a couple pills that night, telling me

to go to bed. And they came in, I was still awake, I had my back towards 'em. And they came in there and started having sex and then—I'll never forget it—he tried to get on top of me. I was moving a lot, you know, and my mom said—I'll never forget it—she said, "Don't hurt her." So I got out of the bed, and I started screaming, yelling, and ran away. And the cops found me and took me back there. I started dealing with the abuse like, "Maybe this is just how my life's supposed to be."

Jaden described similarly horrific experiences:

I was adopted when I was seven. I moved to Florida, and I was so happy 'cause I just felt like I was free, like I didn't have to get abused anymore and all that stuff. Because I went through all kinds of abuse—every abuse you can think of, I went through it. I mean, I went through some gruesome stuff—some *dirty* stuff. I mean, I'm not just talking about sexual, mental, and physical abuse—there was some other stuff I had to do, which I really don't want to talk about over tape, but . . . when I was adopted I was just like so happy and said, "Yes. Thank you. Finally." I didn't know God then, but I knew there was a God, and I thanked God.

When the women I interviewed talked about the abuse they had experienced, statements like "That really messed me up, and I'm just now getting over it" and "I've never been the same since" often followed their stories. Such statements demonstrate the ability of physical experiences to take root in the psyche, producing lasting effects (Bolton et al. 2004). For some women, the effects were evident early. For example, Lisa said, "My first addiction was stealing. I was about six or seven when I started. I was about five when I first started being abused. I started stealing at six and seven to—I don't know, it just made me feel better when I took something that wasn't mine. I kept on stealing for years and years."

For other women, the effects of abuse manifested themselves much later. Linking her childhood abuse to choices she made in adulthood,

Natalie said: "I feel like if the people that are the abusers could see what they're doing to their victims, that would definitely probably curb a lot of abuse. . . . You know, you're having less women that are hurting, so maybe there would be less drug use, less prostitution. I mean, obviously that's not going to stop everything, but it's like, in my case, I wish my stepmother could see how she hurt me."

Natalie's claim that childhood abuse was a precursor to her later propensity for addiction and her involvement in prostitution is corroborated by a fairly large body of evidence suggesting a relationship between the two. Still, the claim that most women in the sex trade have been physically, sexually, or emotionally abused at some time prior to their entering the industry is highly contested. Both because this is a difficult claim to track, and because it seems to promote the idea that participation in sex work is the result of some kind of pathology, pro-sex activists are particularly averse to it. What we do know is that the younger the woman when she enters into sex work, the more likely she is to have been abused. For young adults (mostly "transition age"—that is, eighteen to twenty-two years old) who enter into prostitution, the rates of abuse are staggering. One study of 361 street-involved youth (mean age twenty-two) in Canada found that 73 percent had experienced physical abuse, 32.4 percent had experienced sexual abuse, 86.8 percent had experienced emotional abuse, and 93 percent had experienced emotional neglect (Stolz et al. 2007). Hilary Surratt et al. (2004) and Eloise Dunlap et al. (2002) reported that street-based sex workers experience a cycle of violence involving early experiences with sexual abuse, abuse at work, and abuse in the context of private adult relationships. For men who enter sex work—typically young men—the rates of childhood abuse are even higher (Dilorio, Hartwell, and Hansen 2002; Vanwesenbeeck 2001; Zierler and Feingold 1991). These figures agree with those in other, similar studies of involvement in sex work and childhood abuse (Vaddiparti et al. 2006; West, Williams, and Siegel 2000); however, they do not conclusively demonstrate that involvement in sex work is caused by previous sexual abuse (Nandon, Koverola, and Schludermann 1998; Vanwesenbeeck 2001). That said, it is important to note the prevalence of abuse and to consider that its existence may influence how people regard their own bodies (Dunlap et al. 2002).

ADDICTION

In addition to abuse, the presence and availability of alcohol and drugs was often part and parcel of chaotic family situations. Six of the women I interviewed were using drugs on a regular basis by the time they were twelve. Kathleen, who was nine when her father died in a jail fire, remembers being high at his funeral. Her drug use started the earliest of all the women I interviewed: she drank moonshine for the first time when she was five and smoked marijuana for the first time when she was six. Demetria, who was drinking frequently by the time she was twelve, smoked marijuana for the first time when she was thirteen, snorted powder cocaine for the first time when she was fourteen, and was dealing at the age of fifteen. Linda began stealing from her father's liquor cabinet when she was in the sixth grade. Sasha, whose mother died when she was thirteen, was raised by her siblings and enjoyed the lack of authority, saying it allowed her to spend most of her time using. About her early teenage years, she said, "I pretty much just drank and partied and had kids. My sisters kept my kids all the time. They basically picked up the pieces."

Members of the Magdalene community link early drug and alcohol use to early exposure and modeled behavior (typically by addicted family members) and question whether or not the use of illicit substances at an early age qualifies as a "choice." Although none of my participants reported being forced or even overtly coerced to take their first drink or smoke their first joint, the range of choices presented by their primary caregivers and others in their immediate environments presented few other options. Apart from the six participants who were using drugs regularly by the age of twelve, the majority of the women I interviewed (eleven of nineteen) began using when they were between the ages of thirteen and seventeen. Only two began using after the age of eighteen. For those who started using as teenagers, drugs and alcohol were often characteristic of the environment long before they started using. However, the women who began using as teenagers and young adults credited friends and boyfriends for introducing them to the substances that would later become their constant companions, as in Natalie's case:

> I graduated from high school, I moved out of my parents' house, I got my own place. I was able to take care of myself. I worked. Worked two jobs at times . . . to make sure that I could take care of myself so that I wouldn't have to go back to my family's house. Or go back to my family. Or ask my family for help, because I didn't want to do that. So during that time, when I was about twenty-one years old, I met my son's father, and we jumped right into a relationship. We'd moved in together and that's where the heavy drugs were introduced to me. Prior to that, you know, I had done marijuana and alcohol and some pills and things like that. . . . He was a crack cocaine addict. He had been clean for a couple of years when I met him, but we had been together for about six months and he relapsed. So, at first, I was like, "You can't be in my life. I can't have that," and I would kick him out and we would break up, and then we would get back together and we would break up, and get back together, and he would promise to be clean and this and that and so during all this time, we were together for about three years before I got pregnant with our son, so when I became pregnant, he really straightened up. You know, he cleaned up. We were both working, and saving our money. We got married, which probably wasn't the best of ideas, but we did, we got married. And, everything seemed to be normal. An all-American little family. But when my son was about a year old, my husband relapsed on crack cocaine, and I was just devastated, you know? 'Cause there I am with this baby, and I needed support. I didn't need to be dealing with that, so, it was kind of like, if you can't fight 'em, join 'em. And I fought and I fought and I fought so much to try to keep him clean and keep him off of drugs that I just kind of got sucked into the whole lifestyle.

Natalie's determination to leave home and stay independent of her parents as soon as she was able was a theme common among the women I interviewed.

LEAVING HOME

Most of the women at Magdalene described being rebellious as teen-agers. Certainly, rebellion is a normal part of adolescent development even in the healthiest families. For these women, however, rebellion frequently led to more abuse, and the stifling nature of the environments in which they lived made them desperate for something and someplace different. Ten women reported leaving their families as teenagers. Most report that leaving home was at first an experience of adventure and freedom. Tiffany, for example, ran away from her family in California when she was seventeen, heading for the farthest place she could imagine—Rhode Island. She hitchhiked all the way to Nashville before she got stuck:

> I was hitchhiking in a truck, and I'd be let off at some exit, and then
> I'd get back in another truck, and so on. Anyways, this one truck
> driver, he was an Indian and it was his birthday, and so we went
> into the bar at the truck stop, and . . . for celebrating his birthday we
> were going to have a six-pack of Budweiser. Well, I hadn't had no
> drugs in like three weeks, so some guy come in there with a big ole
> bag of weed and said, "Would you like to come outside with me?"
> I've been here ever since. Honestly. [*laughs*]

Other women, such as Lisa, left home through somewhat more conventional means:

> I got married just to get out of the house. I got married at fourteen,
> but it only lasted a couple years. I was so young; I didn't know
> how to be a wife. We got divorced when I was sixteen. And then I
> started—my mom's been married seven times—I started doing my
> mom's cycle. I started, you know, going, always wanting to be with
> a man. No matter what. So I met this one guy, his name was Gary.
> We lived together for a little while. And then I met William. And we
> stayed together for a little while. And all this time I was using drugs.
> Well, the first time I used drugs was when I was sixteen. When I met
> Gary. I wanted to fit in. So, I started using. . . . I was using heroin,

speed, cocaine—you know, whatever was going on. I started being
dependent on the drugs. And on the men. And then at twenty-one—
no, nineteen—I got married again to my son's father. At nineteen I
got married, and then at twenty-one I had a baby. I quit using when
I was pregnant, and nine months after, I had my son. And then
when I was about twenty-two I got divorced and started using again.

For many women at Magdalene (and elsewhere), men were the
way out of unpleasant family situations. Unfortunately, women often
left abusive families only to find themselves in new abusive relationships. One woman lived with a series of men who each beat her badly
enough to send her to the hospital. Another woman told me about a
boyfriend who pinned her down and stole her false teeth whenever
she called the police to report abuse. If the police took him to jail, he
would take her teeth with him. Another woman talked about a boyfriend who threw her over the railing of a fourth-story balcony when
she told him he couldn't smoke crack cocaine in her apartment. The
police told her that the only reason she survived the fall was because
she herself was high when it happened. As these stories demonstrate,
the violence enacted on the bodies and the psyches of the women at
Magdalene was brutal, and it produced physical and psychological
scars that had lasting effects on their abilities to make choices, form relationships, and act in ways that promoted their own well-being.

Drug Use and Addiction

Each woman reported that her early experiences with drugs had been
positive, exciting, and liberating. Describing her first experience with
marijuana, Kristin said, "I would see my dad drink and I would say,
'I'm never going to drink,' and 'I'm never going to act like that.' And
then I started smoking weed, and I was—whew—I fell in love." Natalie's experience of trying cocaine for the first time was similar: "I did it,
and I loved it. I *loved* it. It took all of my worries and fears away. I could
do anything." Dealing drugs was also a powerful and lucrative experi-

ence for the ten women who reported selling as well as using. Marion said:

> I wanted to make some money and so I started selling marijuana, and you know, smoking the hell out of marijuana, 'cause I had it to do, and I became prestigious in the streets. And then it went from selling weed to selling powdered cocaine, and then I was selling "Ts and Blues" [a heroin substitute]. And then I started selling delottas [Dilaudid pain pills] and I made a whole heck of a lot of money off of delottas.

Marion contrasted dealing with other, legal forms of work, which always came up short: they "just didn't pay me what I was making from the drugs, and so I'd work a job for maybe a few weeks, then I'd stop."

Eventually, though, Marion and others found it difficult to be responsible dealers when they were addicted to the substances intended to bring in a profit: they typically ended up using the drugs they were supposed to be selling, or using the money they earned to buy more drugs for themselves instead of paying their debts to suppliers, landlords, and others.

Many women described drug use as a way not only to feel excitement and power but to numb the pain of traumatic childhood events or abusive relationships, and most of them attributed their propensity for addiction to the families and communities in which they were raised. Others, however, claimed that the link was much more complicated. Shelly recalled a conversation with her cousin, a former addict, in which he urged her to stop using drugs. "You weren't brought up like that," he had said. To which she had replied, "Well, right! But neither were you. And neither were a whole lot of people that are on drugs." Shelly continued, "I don't know if I want to say that it's something that happens or something in your life happens or something that triggers you to do drugs, but there are a lot of different reasons—I honestly believe that—that people start doing drugs."

Regardless of the various, specific reasons that the women at Magdalene began using drugs, their addictions quickly moved toward similar endings. The women reported eventually "settling" on drugs of choice—typically crack cocaine and heroin—that ultimately stopped being agents of power and pleasure and became faceless substances that ruled them as oppressive masters. For many, the process was gradual, but for others, the destructive nature of addiction manifested itself rapidly. Natalie said:

> He and I used pretty steadily on a daily basis for about a year before things really started falling apart. We were behind on our bills, and within about a week's period of time, we lost everything. I lost everything. It was the end of 2005, and my husband got arrested on October 23rd, I lost my job on October the 26th, we got evicted from our apartment on November 1st, and my parents took my son away from me on November 3rd. And so it was just like all of that hit me— bam, bam, bam, bam—and so I just didn't know what to do. And so my parents took my son and they helped me put my stuff in a storage unit. And they tried to help me straighten out, you know, but by this point, I felt like I was so far gone, I didn't know what to do. I didn't want to get clean. I didn't want to have to face all those problems. So that's when I became homeless.

All but two of the women I interviewed were homeless for at least some time during their addiction. The periods of homelessness lasted anywhere from six months to over thirty years. During those stretches of time, women found the means to pay for drugs, food, and temporary shelter by stealing, dealing, prostituting, and sometimes receiving the provision of others, such as service agencies, family members, or friends on the street. During Marion's interview, I asked her what percentage of drug-abusing homeless women she thought were also prostituting. Her estimate was nine out of ten. Although this was a guess informed by Marion's personal experience, large-scale studies confirm that drug addiction (particularly for poor women) and prostitution are closely related (Inciardi and Surratt, 2001). The stories of the other women I interviewed featured this connection as well.

A 1997 study of street-based sex workers in Atlanta revealed that

92.5 percent of the women arrested for prostitution had tested positive for illegal drugs (National Institute of Justice 1998). Another study conducted by a New York organization that has provided health services to sex workers for over twenty years revealed similar levels of drug use among the populations it follows. Of the 144 female sex workers included in the sample, 68.8 percent reported abusing heroin at some point in their lives. Ninety-five percent reported abusing crack cocaine, 84.7 percent powder cocaine, 94.4 percent marijuana, 55.9 percent alcohol, and 40.3 percent benzodiazepines. Ninety-two percent of the women surveyed had used crack cocaine within the last month (Nuttbrock 2004). Researchers note that for sex workers who have active addictions, the relationship between drugs and sex work is not uncomplicated (Durr 2005; Nuttbrock 2004). The need for drug money and the availability of clients among drug-based relationships often means that addiction is the gateway to sex work. Alternately, some women report drug use as a way to numb themselves from the experiences of sex work, and still others report that the environments that support heavy drug use led them to "drift" into the sex trade (Inciardi and Surratt 2001). With this in mind, it is important to note that addiction itself is often a marginalizing and isolating experience. Because of the way that illegal drugs are unequally distributed across population types (Dunlap 2002; Singer 2008), unequal access to effective treatment (Mulia 2002), and the institutional racism that exists in punishment schemes for illicit drug use (Roberts, Jackson, and Carlton-LaNey 2000), addiction is frequently more costly for people of color and those of lower socioeconomic status. Furthermore, addiction in women is often treated differently, both socially and medically, than addiction in men (Mulia 2000; Zerai and Banks 2002). What this means for the women at Magdalene is that the intersections of race, class, gender, sexuality, and life experiences left them particularly vulnerable to the legal and social ramifications that can accompany drug use and abuse. It also suggests that they were especially unlikely to receive appropriate treatment. As a result, the women spent time in prison, lost custody of their children, and learned to sell their bodies to acquire the only things that could satisfy the cravings of addiction.

Prostitution and Life on the Streets

For some women at Magdalene, the journey to the streets of Nashville was little more than stepping out the front door of the homes in which they grew up. Others arrived with a pimp, as runaways, or after years of bouncing around in the foster care system. Jaden, whose story combines these scenarios, was born in Brazil and adopted by an American family, who later kicked her out of the house for "being defiant." She eventually ended up in state custody, where she stayed until she was a legal adult (age eighteen): "Nashville was the last place I landed within the state system. I've been to Memphis. All the little towns and all the cities in Tennessee, I've been there. Foster homes, group homes, just all sorts of different stuff, but Nashville's the last place I landed."

Not long after Jaden arrived in Nashville, she met a man who would eventually become her pimp. She moved into a motel room with him, where they abused various substances and paid for their living expenses through odd jobs, prostitution, and dealing. Sixteen of the nineteen women I interviewed began prostituting to support their addiction. For at least a handful of the women, prostitution was preceded by working as escorts, exotic dancing, or participation in Internet pornography. For most of the women, exchanging sex for drugs with dealers or acquaintances preceded street prostitution. Of the three women who began prostituting for reasons other than addiction, one had run away from home at the age of thirteen and prostituted as a means of survival; two others had been teenagers when they began having sex with neighbors, who in turn paid the girls' mothers and provided extra income for the family. For example, Donna slept with a much older man in her community to help her mother pay rent and utilities when she was unable to make ends meet for their family of seven:

> I'd tell him what would be goin' on at home, or "I've gotta figure out a way to make some money." And I laid with him eventually. We ended up sleeping together, and he would take my mama, I mean, $500 or $600 a time. And my thing was, you're just doing that 'cause you don't want her to know that you're sleeping with your daughter. Man, you're

goin' to go to jail. And I knew it was wrong, and evidently he did too, but I felt like he saved us, our family.

This type of ambivalence toward tricks or the very act of exchanging sex for money was not uncommon. Particularly when they were recalling some of their early experiences with prostitution, women reported feeling a number of emotions, ranging from revulsion to excitement. Kelly said, "I was like really just screwing whoever for whatever. This was the beginning. But, like, it was really exciting to me. Like I felt like I totally had power—like I called the shots." She went on to talk about her experiences with prostitution, saying, "When it comes to absolutely nothing, like you have *nothing*, you can always sell yourself. You don't have to go to work on time, you just—all you have to do is just . . . and it's not hard to find somebody who wants to pay for it. I had an ophthalmologist that traded me contacts for sex. I had a landlord that traded me rent for sex."

When describing some of her first experiences with prostitution, Lisa matter-of-factly outlined a series of events that took her from Nashville to Texas and back, illustrating how easily sex can be used as currency:

> I remember getting in a white pickup and the driver took me
> somewhere, I don't remember where, but I called one of my tricks,
> and he rented a motel for me. And there was this couple—I got
> locked out of my room because the room wasn't in my name,
> and this couple was up on the other floor and they asked me, "Is
> everything OK?" And I said, "No, I'm locked out of my room." So
> they invited me up to their room, and somehow from there they
> talked me into getting in the car with them. They didn't do no dope,
> they didn't do no drugs, but we got stopped in Dallas, and he was
> an escapee from prison. So he got arrested. And that poor girl he
> was with, she was so lost. So we went to a truck stop, I made some
> money, gave her some money for gas and everything, and I talked
> this trucker into letting me travel with him for a while. The truck
> driver brought me to Nashville and dropped me off at another truck

stop, and I made a little bit of money there. I ended up getting with this other trucker and he called over on his CB to another trucker that I needed to go to a certain area, which was Texas, to go to my mom's. So . . . we traveled together for about six months. There were three trucks—Snakeshooter, Moonshiner, and Popcorn. He was really nice. He was actually an angel sent to me. After we got to Texas and he dropped the trailer off, he took me straight to my mom's front door. I'll never forget it. I was about twenty-seven, twenty-eight then. Anyway, I stayed there for just a bit and then somehow I ended up hitchhiking back to Nashville.

Once Lisa returned to Nashville, however, her experiences with prostitution rapidly deteriorated, as did those of every woman I interviewed. Lisa said, "I was seven years out there on the streets, prostituting. Nowhere to go. Nowhere to live. And of course I made some 'acquaintances'—some people that would, you know, I'd pay 'em a little bit of money or sleep with them to stay the night. I was raped twice. I was abused. I had my nose broke twice. So much happened it's just hard to just spit it out."

Multiple studies of sex workers in various locations around the world demonstrate that working conditions make women particularly vulnerable to physical and sexual violence on the job (Sanders and Campbell 2007). Researchers estimate that anywhere from 50 percent to 100 percent of the street-based sex workers in their samples had experienced violence (ibid.). In addition to physical and sexual abuse, the women also fall victim to what some have termed "economic abuse": being robbed, not being paid, or being paid less than the previously agreed-on price for services (ibid.). Street-based sex workers in the United Kingdom are over ten times more likely to die from violence at work than other women their age (Ward, Day, and Webber 1999), and eighty-six sex workers were murdered in the United Kingdom from 1995 to 2005 (Kinnell 2006). In the United States, "standardized mortality rates for sex workers are six times those seen in the general population . . . the highest for any group of women. Death and violence are but a part of a spectrum of physical and emotional morbidity endured" (Goodyear and Cusick 2007, 52). Theorists who believe that violence is inherent to sex work identify prostitution itself as the cause of such violence (Farley and Barkan 1998; Pateman 1988). Others point to stigma, poverty, the general violence of the streets, and the clandestine nature of street-based sex work as the reasons why women are abused (Sanders and Campbell 2007; Vanwesenbeeck 2001).

The violence the women at Magdalene experienced while living on the streets was exacerbated by direct exposure to Nashville's natural and industrial elements (e.g., intense heat, intense cold, car exhaust, and pollution). During a meditation circle at Thistle Farms, Gayle shared that the night before, she had been sitting on the porch at Lena, watching a woman stand on the street corner out in the rain. She recalled the many times she had done the same, and explained how the woman had provided her with a much-needed reminder of how hellish life on the streets could be—wet, cold, and exhausting, with nowhere to go. Discussion about the weather was not uncommon in the circles: women remarked about being happy to be warm when it was cold outside, grateful to be dry when it was raining, and proud to live in a home with air conditioning when the summer temperatures rose to their Tennessee best.

One particularly hot summer, several of the Magdalene staff and residents rented rooms in a motel on Dickerson Road. The hotel was familiar to all the residents—most had been there with tricks too many times to count. This time, however, they were going to "offer love" to women still living on the streets. They invited those women to come in, eat, and take a bath. Some guests asked to stay long enough to take a nap—to sleep in a bed, indoors, in a cool, comfortable place where the risks of rain, robbery, and rape were absent.

I often heard women at Magdalene compare their physical appearances now to when they lived on the streets. For many, physical appearance was a metric for the extreme conditions they had endured. For example, Kayla recounted a morning that has stuck in her mind:

> It's about 2 or 3 a.m., it's pretty cold out, I have on some stretch pants
> that I got from somebody else that I've had on for probably about
> four days, and I have on some pants over the top of the stretch pants

that I've had on probably about four or five days, and I have on a
sweatshirt, and it's dirty and smelly, and I have on a jacket—not a coat,
just a jacket—and I have on a hat.

As she continued describing that morning to me, her words conveyed
both the fear and the all-consuming nature of addiction that many of
the women had experienced:

I walk up Hancock, which is one of the streets in East Nashville, and
at that time of the morning, there are no cars really on that side of the
street. So I really can't see, except for the lights from the vehicles, and
. . . it's real spooky. And every now and then, you'll see the headlights
from a car, and I remember turning to look on the top of the car to see
if it's a police car—if I could see the lights or not, or if it's a trick that's
ridin' down the street. And I remember this one particular morning,
as I was coming up the street, another young lady that has now been
through the program [Magdalene] was coming down the street. And
a lot of times, that time of the morning when it was quiet and no cars
were rolling and it was scary, I would cry. I'd walk and cry, walk and
cry and walk and cry, and I remember this morning, I saw this lady,
and she was crying and walking, too. And we both kind of stopped,
and I had some drugs that morning, and we kind of like, stopped, right
where we met, sat on somebody's steps right in front of the house, and
smoked some crack. And she went on her way and I went on my way.
But how scary and lonely and isolated that felt, and it was during a
time when a young lady had gotten murdered in that area, too, so it
was a real scary time. So that always stands out, . . . how we crossed
each other's paths that morning. And, you know, we were both saying,
"Ain't nobody out here but us," and she was saying, "Yeah, us and
somebody crazy."

Fear of being killed on the streets was common among the women,
and several described near-death experiences resulting from drug violence or abusive tricks. During their time on the streets, the women
were robbed, raped, beaten, stabbed, shot, kidnapped, and pushed out

of cars. They were abused by tricks, dealers, police, and other prostitutes. Similarly, they robbed, stabbed, and shot other people to stay alive, exact revenge, or score the next hit.

For many of the women, life on the streets was ultimately an unending cycle of homelessness, prison, and inpatient treatment centers, none of which seemed to have any kind of permanent effect. Kathleen described her last day on the streets:

> I can remember standing on the side of the street, cussing God, asking God why my life had to be the why it was, why he didn't allow me to die. And I can remember being suicidal, wanting to die. Didn't want to die, but didn't want to live, neither. And I can remember asking him, "If I take this next hit, let me die or send me to jail." And let me say, I found God in the back of the police car. And, staying in jail for thirty-six days, I began to make some decisions. I didn't want to continue to live the life that I was living. And I wanted a way out. And I can remember going to court, asking the judge for some help. And asking him for a long-term program, because I had been in programs before. But I went into them programs to beat the system. Not really wanting to stop. I just wanted the pain to go away. And I was so sick and tired of being sick and tired of myself. I wanted something different.

Women at Magdalene often tell the stories of their last day using—a common practice in many recovery communities. These stories are powerful reminders of the lives they left behind. When boredom, frustration, cravings, or coping with life events threatens to lead to relapse, the memory of life on the streets is often enough to keep a person clean. These stories are also the stories of how the women came to Magdalene, and capture a crucial step in the journey so many women describe as "coming home." Kayla's story includes the metric of physical appearance mentioned earlier in this chapter:

> I remember my last day using. The last time I turned a trick. I got in the car with this guy, and he asked me to have sex with him for money, and I just remember how bad I wanted to say no. I wanted

to say no so much I could barely stand it. But by that time, I was
using against my own will, and I just wanted to numb the pain that
I was feeling from being in the streets and using, and I turned the
trick and I purchased drugs to get high, and the drugs were not
working anymore. They were not numbing the pain. I remember
seeing a friend girl of mine, her name was Shelby, she was in the
program, and when I saw her this time—I used to get high with
her—but when I saw her this time there was something different
about her.[2] She was so pretty and vibrant, she was glowing, and I
asked her where she had been, 'cause I knew she hadn't been on
the streets with me anymore, and she told me about the Magdalene
program. And she began to tell me about how I needed to try this
program, and instantly, for me, it was like—'cause I'd already done
five or six treatment centers—and I said, "No, I don't want to do
another treatment center, they don't work for me." But she began to
tell me how different that Magdalene program was, and I could see
the difference in her. And she went back and she talked to the house
manager and the program staff, and I was allowed to come in.

Lisa recalled how exhausted she felt:

My last day using: I didn't care, I was lost, I had some money, I had
some dope in my pockets, I tore it up, threw the dope away. I was
tired. So I went to a friend's, he's a guy, the first guy who wouldn't
sleep with me. And I went to his house and I said, I want treatment,
I want some help. And he said, "Well, come on. Get some rest.
Take you a shower, get some rest. We'll see what we can do in the
morning." So the next morning, I woke up and he wasn't there, so
I went back to sleep, then he came and woke me up, and said, "My
boss is out here, ready to take you to go get some help." So I got up,
washed my face, went outside, got in the back seat of the boss's car,
and my friend got in the front seat with his boss. His boss turned
around and looked me in the eyes and said, "We're gonna get you
some help." So he took me to McDonald's first, got me something
to eat. No, it was Burger King. And then he, they had trouble

finding this place, but it was like God was just pulling his truck, you know, here, here. And we stopped out front and he said, "This is the place." And I said, "Oh my," you know? I looked at the house and said, "Oh my." And he said, "Well, you want me to go in first? Or you just want to go in?" So his boss—his boss don't even *know* me—comes in and says, "Can I speak to someone?" And Angela, who was here before, said, "No, we don't take people like that," but somehow Miss Sonya seen me, and had grace on me. They took me in that day. You're supposed to be on the waiting list, but I was not. And I thank God every day for that. Just—it's a miracle that I'm here.

For Lisa and Kayla, coming to Magdalene was an easy choice, and once they had made the decision to come, the road to get there was smooth. Other women described the difficulty of deciding to come, and the often heartbreaking transition that occurred when they realized that their need for help was serious enough to trump all other commitments. This was Donna's experience:

I heard about Magdalene through a friend of mine. I supposed to go to Magdalene [on] June 3, 2007, but I didn't go. . . . I wanted to go, but I didn't want to leave my kids, 'cause my mama had said she would take care of all four of my children if I was there to help her. And the judge was OK with that as long as I was being supervised, but hell, I got high at my mama's house. She went to bed before I did, the kids were little—so, it didn't matter. But I done good for a little while—I wasn't using, and so I called Magdalene and told 'em I wasn't coming. Thanks for everything, but I'm not coming. So I was working, I had a car, I was gaining all my stuff back, but then, this last time, I got high and I went out, and within two weeks, if that, it was all *gone*. So I called my friend Patrice who was in NA [Narcotics Anonymous], and I was like, "OK, I'm sorry I can't do it, I need your help. And you said that anytime I want some help you would help me, so . . ." She didn't answer the phone, but I left it on her answering machine. And I still didn't hear nothing. I even called Magdalene's phone, but I didn't hear nothing, didn't hear nothing. And I had gave up—I was like, "Fuck it, I'll handle it the best that I can. Fuck NA, they just talk a bunch of bullshit, the motherfuckers ain't gonna help." I mean all of that. I went through all of that. And then June 10th, 2008, at 9:30 p.m., I got a knock at my mama's door, and it was Shawn, a girl from my neighborhood, and she handed me the phone and it was Patrice, and she said, "You've got fifteen minutes to decide what you want to do," and I was like, "Patrice, there's gonna be some shit. My mama's gonna go off." But she didn't even have to ask me that question—I was ready. I had just gotten through gettin' high when she knocked at the door, and I said, "It's gonna be some shit, my mama's gonna flip out." And there was. So Shawn, Kayla, and Patrice came and got me. And my mom was like, "You just don't want to deal with your kids, you don't want no responsibility, you just want to put it off on everybody else." And I'm like, "Mom, it's not like that. But if I don't get some help, I'm not gonna be good to none of y'all." I heard my kids crying, and my oldest son said to me, "Mama, why did you call them to come get you? We're gonna be OK. We're gonna make it." That hurt. And I was like, "Baby, mama gotta get some help, so I can take care of you better." And he was like, "But you ain't gotta leave!" I will never forget that. I remember that like it was yesterday. He just kept saying, "You ain't gotta go, mama." Oh my God. I didn't think I was going to be able to live through the heartache. The shame. The fear. But then the next day came, and the next day came, and the next day. And I was still alive. I didn't call my mom for like a week 'cause I didn't know what to say to her. But then I talked to Shawn and she was like, "You need to call your mama," you know? So like a week passed and I called her and it was nothin' but love. It wasn't like the night I had left and she was so upset, but she was like, "OK, baby. You gotta do this. You gotta do whatever you can do to get well. And I want you to be able to keep these kids." And . . . it's just been a blessing ever since.

The many debates about prostitution, drug use, and the lifestyles that leave women on the streets include disagreements about freedom, responsibility, and choice. Knowing whether or not a woman chooses to be on the streets—whether or not she's responsible for her own distress—seems to be the divining rod used to determine where to cast blame. And being able to blame someone—parents, family members, neighbors, boyfriends, or the women themselves—is the tool many people want in order to chart a course of action regarding what should be done about the "problem" of prostitution and drug use. At Magdalene House, the questions of blame and guilt are asked less often, and the members of the community stress the importance of a different kind of choice: regardless of why or how a woman gets to the streets, they say, she should be able to choose to leave.

CHAPTER 3

The Story of One

When I think about the women who I see coming into
this program, I think that, well, while they have all had
horrendous childhoods filled with abuse and neglect,
and have ended up addicted and prostituting—you
know, everybody's story is going to be pretty different.
And once you get to the point where they're all victims
of abuse, women who've been oppressed, women who
need to be freed, prostitutes—once you lump 'em all
together, I get uncomfortable.
        —Lynn, Magdalene House staff member

B ECAUSE NARRATIVES OF ADDICTION and recovery are so
   often individual stories of personal failure and triumph, one of my
goals in writing this book is to help connect these individual stories—
their accounts of abuse, despair, poverty, healing, hope, and change—
to the broader systems, environments, and relationships that created
them. I write about these things to draw attention to the need for better systems, environments, and relationships rather than reformed individuals. Human flourishing will be limited in important ways until
we do a better job of shaping the laws, economic practices, and social
beliefs that form the contexts in and through which humans exist. At
the same time, as Lynn's words illustrate, something is lost in talking
only about systems and inequalities, or even in talking about the gen-
eralized experiences of a small group of people. The world around us
takes root in our very beings and shapes us (and in turn is shaped by

us) in ways that are at least a little bit different for each person, a reality
of which I was reminded often during my time at Magdalene House.
Whether the differences and similarities are the result of genetic fabric,
creative design, or social ideologies (or all or none of these forces) is
beyond the scope of this book. What *is* within the scope of this book is
presenting the women with whom I worked in the most humane way I
know how; among other things, they embraced me with overwhelming
hospitality, and they were brave and kind enough to share their stories
with me. In the interest of honoring the many "pretty different" stories
of the women at Magdalene, this is the story of one, in her own words.

My name is Marion and I'm forty-seven years old, and I'm
grateful that I've made it this far. Thinking back, I think about
growing up in the house with my parents. I had both my parents growing up and they both worked two jobs, and I was the
oldest of three and I was responsible for everything: cleaning
the house, making sure that my brother and sister were doing what they were supposed to do, and, Mom, she kept us in
church all the time. And I hated church, I hated that I had to
do everything, and that I had to make sure we were at church
and everything. Sunday morning, Sunday night, Tuesday
night, Wednesday night, the orientation class for whatever was
going on that week, then on Fridays, praise sessions, just being in church all the time, and I felt like I never learned anything. Like, . . . what was the purpose? You know? And, I think
like around the sixth grade, I became interested in boys and I
wanted a boyfriend, Davis, and of course my mom and daddy
said no, but I was always curious—curious about the boys and
curious about hanging out in the neighborhood, but my mom
never allowed us to be outside after dark—we had to be inside.
And I remember being in the Girl Scouts and going camping
and stuff that the little girls in our neighborhood never got to do.
I got to do some things that other kids didn't get to do, but my
mom was so strict, and she meant it about church.

So when I was in the ninth grade, I met this boy that was in
the eleventh grade and I fell in love. And, later in 1979, I mar-

ried this guy because I had gotten pregnant. And so I was going
into the tenth grade and I had to drop out of school because I
stayed sick all the time, and later on that year in September, we
ran away and got married in a courthouse and I was just like,
Oh, that was *freedom*, coming out of my mom's house and my
mom's strict rules where I couldn't do anything other than be
at home and take care of my brother and sister. So I married
this guy and we moved in public housing on Shelby Avenue—
Casey Homes. And I thought was he my air—I was so in love.
I was raised to believe that the man was the head of the house
and what he says goes, so I was very submissive to my husband.
He eventually became very controlling—he became an abuser.
He never allowed me to be outside if he wasn't there. When he
came home, he would check me—my vagina—to be sure that
nobody had been there and I had not been having sex and all
this crazy stuff, and he used to smoke weed a lot. We used to
fight and he used to beat me up all the time—like if I went on
an errand with my mom, when she brought me back, he would
beat me up because he thought she had taken me to meet
somebody. He was just insanely jealous. He really controlled
everything about me, and I had my first son at that time, and
I used to literally think that he was going to kill me. The last
time that he beat me, I was in the tub, and you know how those
old-fashioned bras that they used to have in the seventies had
the things that you would tighten them up with and they would
leave marks on your shoulders? Well, he said that they were passion marks, and said I was cheating on him, so he hit me and
knocked me into the brick wall—you know in the projects all
the walls is made of brick—and he knocked me out. And when
I came to, he was on the floor crying, saying he's not gonna hit
me again, and on and on. And I just realized that he was eventually going to kill me, because this happened every other day, if
not every day. And I was thinking about my son, and thinking he
was gonna kill me, and he was gonna kill my son. The next day,
I got up enough courage to stand up to him and told him that
I was leaving—one of us was leaving. And he's like, "Nobody's

leaving," and I'm like, "One of us is leaving, it's either you or it's me," and I bluffed him—I lied because I was just so tired of the ass-whoopin's—I bluffed him and said, "Well, if we're going to fight, we might as well get it over with because my dad's on his way over to pick me up." My dad wasn't on his way, but I said that. And, the punk left, you know? The punk left. He was not a man at all.

After he left—I had come out of a strict home environment with my mom and my dad, and I jumped into an even stricter household with my husband—and so when he left, it was just like, "Man, I'm fixin' to see what's up!" You know? And there was this street—I lived on South Seventh in East Nashville and the street behind me was South Eighth, and I was never allowed to go on that street, so of course I wanted to go see what the big deal was. There was this store up there and everybody was hanging out in the street, and it was just like, man, this is *live*, you know? It looks like they're having a good time, and all kinds of men, and the girls—everyone was just hanging out. I started hangin' out with one of my neighbors that lived behind me, started smoking weed, and we went to the store up there one day and I met this guy. I saw this guy and, God, he was just *shining*. He looked really good, and his name was Leon. I was just like, "Who is that nigger?" I was like, "Dang, I wouldn't mind getting with him." And what happened, he ended up coming to my house to take me to dinner, and for the first time in my life that I could remember, I had fun—I learned how to have fun. I learned how to laugh, and he treated me like nobody's ever treated me. He furnished my whole apartment. I lived in the projects, but it looked like I lived in a nice apartment, and he took care of my son, he took care of me. I never had to ask for anything, it was just there. Eventually, my curious mind said, "He doesn't work. So where is he gettin' the money?" He told me—showed me—what he was doing. He was selling marijuana and Demerol—that was in the eighties, about '81. Anyway, he showed me what he was doing and how he was doing it, and so I started selling. I was in the game, you know? I sold marijuana, cocaine, pills—back then, they called that "the poor man's high"—then I learned how to cook the powdered cocaine up into freebase, into crack. I didn't understand why people would come and buy all of this crack, and started to wonder, "What does it make you feel like?" And again my curious mind got the better of me, so I tried it. I didn't understand it because I didn't think that it did anything to me, but it must have, because months later I was like, "I need to smoke some." I needed it. I wanted it. And I kept smoking and selling and from '81 to '84, I was just rollin'—selling my drugs, making money, going different places, and in '84, I got pregnant with my second son, so I slowed down a bit, and then in the middle of '85, I got pregnant with my third son. Not long after that, their father died in a drug deal that went bad. After that, I was just lost, you know? This man that I had met—not Leon, his name was Timothy—when he died, it was like my whole world just collapsed, and I went into using more and more crack, and I always said that that's what I always would do to make my money.

What happened was I ended up using more of my product than I should have, and I started being careless with the money, and ended up using the money to buy drugs just to get high. I remember thinking to myself at the beginning of my using that I would probably just smoke weed and drink my wine until I die. I didn't know that I was speaking a curse on myself—because that's what I now believe it was—and it escalated from the marijuana to the pink Champale to the Wild Irish Rose to the powdered cocaine in the joints, to the crack, and then the crack became *everything* to me. I had always said, "Honey, I would never be a prostitute," you know? "I would never sell my body," and "How do women do that? That's just nasty! Why would you do that?" Only to find myself doing that very thing.

The first time I did it, I didn't have to have sex. I was asked to go as an escort to this banquet with a lawyer, and he's still around today, and I love him. I love him because he was not abusive; he was just a gentleman, what I thought a man was supposed to be anyway. He bought me this beautiful dress, some-

thing that I had never had before, and he took me to the Hyatt
Regency downtown, and I walked into this room full of people
with him. I felt so out of place, but I thought, "Wow, what an
opportunity to be around all these people." And he was so proud
to have me as his date, you know, and at the end of the night,
he gave me $300 and I thought, "He wants to have sex, right?"
But he never said any of that. He just said, "Thank you—hope
you have a good rest of the night," and sent me home. I was
like, "Dang, if that's what prostitution is, then I can do that." So
it started out that I went to work for an escort service, and then
from the escort service I ended up in this little dive on Dickerson Road, dancing, and from there I ended up literally getting
tricks off the street. And it was because of using more and more
of the crack—that's a hellified drug right there—and I began to
leave my sons more and more. It started out that I was escorting
and prostituting because I made more money from them than I
was from selling drugs, and it was that way because I was using
the drugs. So I said, "OK, I can do this and pay my bills and take
care of my sons." It didn't end up working that way. I ended up
leaving my sons—my oldest son was like eleven or twelve at the
time—and I had begun to do the same thing to them that I felt
my mom had done to me. I left him at home to take care of his
two brothers and he became the parents. I was out gettin' high
and messin' up my life. So that went on from '81 all the way to
'96. I lost custody of my children in '89—thank God that my
parents took them—but that didn't stop me. It depressed me,
it made me angry, because I couldn't see that I wasn't being a
good mother. I thought that as long as they were in school and
they had a roof over their heads, that everything was fine, but it
wasn't. And so my parents took custody of them and I went full
blown into the streets—the prostitution, the getting high, being
mad at the world, feeling like the love of my life had died, and
if he hadn't died, then my life wouldn't be like this, and oh my
mother's just turning my children against me, and just blam-
ing everybody and everything else for me not getting or seeking
help. And I stayed out there for years. From '81 to '96, in and

out of jail, going back to the streets, and swearing, "this time, as soon as I got out of jail, I'm going home." But I never made it home.

I REMEMBER THE YEAR that I had prayed my last prayer, and I'm telling you, I hated going to church, and I believed that I never learned anything. But I was thinking about that year, and I was walking down one of the main strips in East Nashville, Meridian Street—I was going to Dickerson Road—and I remember my mama's voice coming in my head and saying, "Marion, pray. Pray." I remember thinking, "What am I going to pray for?" I had been raised in the Church of Christ and they said that if you do anything outside of the church, or that your mom or daddy hadn't taught you, then you were going to hell. And I had had a baby out of wedlock, my marriage didn't work out, I was selling drugs, I was selling myself, and so, *hell*, what the hell am I going to pray for? But I kept hearing her in my head, saying to pray. I began to pray because, at that time, I felt like I was going to die on those streets. I thought that I wasn't going to be able to see my sons again—that I wasn't going to be able to be whole, you know? All I really wanted was to go home and be a mother to my children. I didn't want to smoke any more dope, I didn't want to turn one more trick, but I was caught up and didn't know any way out. Throughout that whole time, I believe that God was sending me people that would come and say, "Girl, you don't need to be out here, you need to go home," or my mom saying, "You need help. You need treatment or something," and I was like, "I don't need no treatment. I can stop when I want to stop." But one day, I realized I couldn't.

I began to pray and I began to ask God, "If you're real, do something. You see I'm down here struggling." But I hadn't ever experienced God, really, so I'd start out praying, but then I'd end up cussing God out. I was just like, "You motherfucker, you're sittin' up there on your high throne . . ." but, now, let me say, I'm not trying to justify it, but I had a crack pipe in my hand, and I was hittin' the crack pipe and cussin' God, I was hittin' my crack pipe and I was cussin' God, and I was like, "Do something!"

I was crying and asking God to look inside of me, and I walked down to Dickerson Road and this police car come flyin' by. He did a U-turn in the street, and he was just like, "What are you doing out here?" You know, it was like two o'clock in the morning, and I was like, "What the fuck do you think I'm doin' out here?" I had an attitude, you know, and he said, "You got any warrants on you?" And I was like, "I probably do, why don't you go check?" And so he goes to the car and he's got a partner in the car and they ran my name, and I had a warrant. And he comes back and says, "Well, you've got an outstanding warrant, but I'll tell you what, I'm gonna let you go." And I was like, "No! What the hell? Why are you—?" Because I wanted to get *off the street*, you know? So I told the police officers, "If you don't take me to jail, man, if you do not take me on in, I'm gonna make you. It's cold, and I want to get off the street." I was tired and I was thinking I was gonna die, and I was afraid they weren't going to take me to jail. I told him I was gonna bust his damn windows out. I was like, "If you do not take me in, I am bustin' your windows out." Then they start in with, "Oh, you fuckin' crazy. Get your ass off the street." So I bent down, picked up some bricks and some rocks and started throwing them at their car, and the cop was like, "Are you motherfuckin' crazy?" And I said, "Are *you* motherfuckin' crazy?" And they came out and they grabbed me all up, handcuffed me, and threw me in the car, and I was so *happy*. I was so happy to be going to jail. I was just like, "Thank you, God!" You know? And then I started laughing—they probably thought I was mental or something—but I started laughing because I realized that God had answered my prayer. And when I got to the jail, I was happy. I hated getting quailed, but I was ready to get quailed, let them take my blood, do the TB test— I'm ready to get to the unit, you know? I'm ready to start my life.

What I thought was freedom was really bondage. It was really a series of being in the streets, learning how to sell the drugs that were killing people and myself, putting myself in bad situations with the prostitution, losing my children, losing the lifestyle that I had been brought up in, and ending up in a dark place that I thought that I was never going to get out of. Being consumed by that crack. That was bondage. It was like I had sold my soul for the crack. "If you just give me one more hit, then you can do anything to me." I allowed so many things to happen to me. And there were a lot of things that I didn't allow, but that happened anyway—the rapes and all of that. And, then there was the bondage of believing the lie that "this is it"—that I've gone too far. Only to remember God—not really believing that this entity would even hear me, but I tried and I opened my mouth and I asked for help out of that dark hole that I had dug for myself. When I was delivered that day and I was taken to the penitentiary, I saw for the first time that I was free—that I didn't have to go back, and I didn't want to go back, and I was free.

When I got to the unit, you know, people I knew—people I'd been in and out of jail with were there and I saw this woman I knew from the streets, and she was in jail, and we started reminiscing. We were like, "Girl, dang. We cut up, didn't we?" We were talking about getting high and how we done scammed some dude, and she was like, "Well, I'm getting' out tomorrow." And I've been in that place, you know? Been in the place of just wantin' to be back out, rippin' and runnin', but this time was different. This time, I was like, "Well, I'm not trying to get out. Whatever they're going to give me, I want to do the time." Which ended up being eighteen months that last time. I went through this program called "Chances." Isn't that ironic? Chances. I graduated that program, and I took a course in business that they offered at the prison. I got my little certificate for going through that, and both of those business teachers were very spiritual. It was like God was just placing people in front of me to help draw me to him, and to let me know that I could have a life.

When I went up for parole, they gave it to me, and I was happy about the parole, but I was scared to death at the same time. Because, I mean, for *years*, I was going in and out of jail, and I had lost everything—I had lost my boys, most of all—but I had lost everything. And I was just so afraid of going back to the streets, wanting to go home like I did every single time, and not making it. I didn't want to leave—I didn't want to leave prison, 'cause it was like that was my safety net. That was my safe haven. And I was just like, "What am I gonna do? What am I gonna do?" By this time, of course, my mother or my father didn't believe shit I had to say. They were like, "You've said it all before, you've tried to do it all before, only to leave again." And my children were so happy whenever I came around, but their question mark was always, "When is she gonna disappear?" So I was like, "I don't know. I don't know what am I gonna do." I'm telling you, my mom's voice came in my head and said, "Marion, have you prayed? Pray." And I thought about that and I went and I prayed and I asked God to help me again. And I thanked him for bringing me to CCA [Corrections Corporation of America]. Then I said, "But if I walk outside of these doors, I don't know what I'm gonna do. I don't know what I'm gonna do."

This is the story of all of us. We go in for three, seven, maybe thirty days, we come back out and it's the same damn thing. And, I had such an addiction to crack that I didn't even want to see the dope anymore. I was afraid to see dope. So I went to my counselor's office, and we were talking about my parole plan. I was telling her I was scared. Right then, her phone rang, and when her phone rang it was one of the girls that I had been incarcerated with. She was just calling in to check on the girls, and keeping connected, and she asked to speak to me. My counselor let her talk to me, and she was like, "What are you doing when you get out? I heard you made parole." I said, "I don't know what I'm doing, but I'm scared, and I want to go home." She asked, "Well, is that a good place for you?" I said, "Well, that's where my kids are." And she was just like, "Well, I found this place, it's a halfway house." I was like, "A halfway house? What is that?" She said, "Well, they help you get into treatment. Do you want to do some more treatment?" I was

like, "I just want to do anything so that I don't have to go back
to the streets." She started telling me about this place she called
"Magdalene." I asked what I had to do to get in, and she gave
me the program director's number. Finally, she said, "Girl, I'm
just telling you, this is the place you need to be. All the hos is
over here." Then she told me this woman I knew named Charla
was there, and she said Pamela and Julia were there too, and
she said, "Girl, it is nice. It is really nice." I said, "But all the
girls over there, what are you all doing?' And she said, "This is a
place just for us hos." I was just like, "Oh hell no. I'm not trying
to prostitute anymore." And she says, "No—they just want you
to come and just start living your life, you know?" So I asked,
"Well, who's over it?" She said, "Girl, it's this priest, her name is
Becca." And I was like, "Oh hell fuckin' no. I'm not fixin' to go
anywhere that's got a priest. What do you gotta do? Do you gotta
go to like Mass or something? Do you gotta go say Abba Fathers,
and a thousand Hail Marys? What do they want you to do?" She
just laughed at me, and she said, "Girl, you just need to come
on over here. We doin' good. We just doin' *good*." And so she
gave me the number and I called the program director back
then who was named Elizabeth, and she said, "Yes, we have a
bed," and she sounded like somebody that—just, I don't know.
She was just too nice. Too. Nice.

When I got out of prison, I would not leave that property.
I'm telling you I was scared to death. My sister came and picked
me up, and she took me to Magdalene's house, the first house
over on Park. When I saw that house I was like, "This is not it.
This is not it!" You know? I guess in my mind I was thinking
about a boarding house or something, but it was just beautiful
on the outside, and the yard—it had a yard, and a fence, a big
porch. I was just like, "This can't be it!" The next thing I know,
Charla and Pamela and RayAnn and Julia all come running out
the door and they were clean. You know, they were *clean* and
they were *glowing*, and I was like, "Wow," you know, and I was
like, "Man, y'all look like new money. Whatever y'all doin', I
want some of it." We were all just huggin', cryin'. I walked into

this house and it was beautiful on the inside, too, and it was just like — it was home. I tell this part of the story in particular because it did remind me of home. And to think where I had just come from — jail — and before jail it was the streets and empty houses and motels and in the alleys — sleeping in the alleys and literally being in the streets. I walked through that house and there was furniture in there, and a bed, a beautiful bed, and they had dishes in the kitchen. I started crying. They were laughing and picking with me, and I was just like, "Do y'all know, man? We just come from cookin' dope up in spoons and jars and stuff." On the streets, there wasn't no dishes or nothing, you know? There wasn't nothing like this.

My mind was still kind of saying, "What's the deal? What is the deal?" I was in that prostitution mentality — if you're giving me something, it means you want something. I was walking through there and they were talking about being there for two years, and not having to pay rent or any bills and these people just wanted us to relax and rest and decide what we wanted to do with our lives, and I was like, "Huh-uh. Huh-uh. There's something up." You know what I'm saying — who in their right mind is going to pay rent for me? For two years. I mean, who? They want something. You know? But I never found what it was, except for me to get my life together.

When I first came to Magdalene, they bought me clothes 'cause I had no clothes, and Elizabeth had taken me to buy a coat. It was getting cold, so we went to East Nashville, and that was my old stomping ground. She went down Trinity Lane, and I was like, "Oh my God!" I started freaking out, you know? I was like, "You've gotta get me out of here!" I was laying down in her car and she was like tripping out, "What's wrong?" My stomach was doing flips and I was having butterflies and I started shaking and I started crying and I was like, "Elizabeth, you gotta get me out of here, you gotta get me out of here." In the beginning, I couldn't even be in the environment, you know? I couldn't even be in the environment 'cause it was just like it was pullin' me or something. I was so afraid that I was gonna see somebody, or I

would want to get out of the car, or *something*. But I think back
to Elizabeth and how she must have felt dealing with us. It's like
when I first heard her on the phone I thought, "Gah, she sounds
so corny," you know? She was just too nice. She was just so
pleasant. I just thought, "There's something to that. Nobody can
be that nice." She's saying stuff like, "Oh, sweetie, baby, honey,"
you know? But I think back to how defiant and rebellious I was
with that woman. I mean, to the point of even calling her a
prejudiced bitch. I think about her a whole lot of days, and I just
want to call her and tell her, "I am so sorry!" [*laughs*] Because
she was in some fresh water with us. Didn't know what was in
it, you know? Dealing with us five women from the streets. She
had no clue. And neither did Becca, but she had big love in
spite of it. Becca will still say to me sometimes, "You gotta learn
to love tough people." Or I'll be dealing with someone or something and she'll tell me, "That's your spiritual teacher." And
when I think back to Elizabeth, I wonder, "Did she think we
were her spiritual teachers? Did she have that?" 'Cause we gave
her hell. And it was just her dealing with us most of the time.
Then when Becca would come around it would be like, "OK,
mama's home. We gotta get it in line."

I guess I went through Magdalene for maybe two or three
months before I ever met Becca. I had never seen this lady priest
that they were talking about, and then one Saturday, Charla
was babysitting for Becca, and I came out of my bedroom and I
was like, "Charla, whose baby is that?" . . . She said, "Oh, that's
Becca's baby." He went through the hall and this girl picked
him up and then Charla said, "Have you met Becca?" I said
"No. Where is she at?" And the girl with the baby was Becca,
you know? But she was not what I expected. Not at all what I expected. I used to just watch Becca when she was around, and I
learned so much about me from watching her. She's just simple.
You know what I'm saying? She's simple. And she's full of love,
and she preaches God's grace and his mercy. I don't know every
detail of her life growing up, but her trials seem just like mine.
Even though she wasn't on the streets and she wasn't in the

dope houses, she still understood. I came to Magdalene and somebody finally understood. She understood what the pain was like, what the struggle was like. And she reached her hand out and it was just like she was saying, "You don't have to be afraid." Plus all the people that support her. That supported me. You know, when I was out on the streets, I—we all—believed that nobody cared, that people thought like I thought: that prostitutes were the scum of the earth.

I remember when I was living at Magdalene, my brother had me some cards made and they said, "Women in recovery, we do recover." They had my number on them—the Park Avenue house number on it. So every time I'd see somebody I knew from the streets, I'd give them one of my cards, and at two and three o'clock in the morning, the phone would start ringing, and my housemates would be going, "Oh, Marion, the phone is for you! You got people calling you at two and three o'clock in the morning—what's wrong with you?!" It would always be one of the girls from the street saying, "OK, what do I need to do?" And "I don't want to do this no more. Can I come to where you are?" And I would go to Becca and I would be like, "We gotta do something—they're calling me." I would be in trouble with the other girls in the house, of course, because the phone would be ringing, and I would just be like, "These are our sisters and they want off the street. Don't they deserve a chance?" That would be my defense—I would tell Becca, "We gotta. . . ." And she was like, "Marion, what do you want to do?" And I was like, "I don't know! Can we put 'em in a hotel?" Not thinking, really, but just so excited about somebody else wanting to come off the streets. We tried the hotel thing, not really thinking about the mentality of the prostitute or the drug addict, and it turned out they were gettin' high and turnin' tricks in the hotel. So that didn't work. [*laughs*] But I kept after it, and several years later, Becca found some grant money and said, "This is what we're going to do. We're going to create an outreach, so you go ahead and think up some ideas for what you want to do." So we started going out to the different strips where the women are—Dicker-

son Road, Murfreesboro Road—we've done one right up here
on this corner before the houses were built. We would take and
serve lunch, give clothes—the first one, we did pedicures and
manicures and we had toiletry bags and all kind of information
about treatment and the different halfway houses and our recovery home, and we never tried to get people to do something they
weren't ready for. It doesn't work like that. But we just loved
'em and helped 'em take care of their bodies just a little bit, you
know? We just said, "When you're ready . . ."

I loved the outreaches, and I still love them even though
we don't do 'em as much, but I love it because I get to share
freedom with people. And freedom is knowing that I don't have
to pick up another piece of crack. Now I can be around it and
it doesn't affect me, but remember at the beginning, I didn't
want to see—I couldn't even see it. I couldn't even be in the
neighborhood. But today I can go back to the environment
and do an outreach. That's freedom. In the beginning, it was
still like I was in bondage and I did not want to be back on the
streets. But today, I'm free to walk in this neighborhood. I used
to get high on this corner. I used to get high on that corner.
[*points*] On that one. [*points*] On that one. Lena used to be the
dope house that everybody came to and we'd be in the back
bedrooms and the back and the front. We'd give a hit to get in,
and sit back there and just get high, turn a trick, whatever. This
whole neighborhood, all the way from Mt. Nebo on up to Forti-
eth, the projects was drug infested, and it still is, but I'm so glad
we're in the middle of it. Because guess what, we get to be the
lights in the neighborhood. You know what I'm saying? Because
the women that walk these corners, walk these streets, they
come and they ask, "What is this?" And, "How can I get help?"
Some of the guys, the dope dealers, come around and say they
"got a sister," or "gotta friend," and "can you help them?"

You know, at the beginning, people were like, "You're gonna
build a recovery house right there? On that corner? Do y'all
know what y'all doin'?" And it turned out to be a great idea.

That's freedom—from everything that could hold you down in the drug world, the street life—you know, being able to be sit smack dab in the middle of it and go out and just say, "Hey, *your* change is coming." It ain't in your time, it ain't in my time—for real—it's in God's time. A lot of the women who have been through the program came from this very neighborhood: Terry, Valerie, Pamela, Rochelle, Charlene, Charnita, Vanessa, Melvina—there are others. Anyway, several women from this neighborhood have come through Magdalene. So it's a sanctuary, right in the middle of a drug-infested neighborhood, and I'm proud of that. Proud to be a part of it.

A couple of months ago, this guy, he had just gotten out of jail, and came walking by and said, "What the hell? What is this place? When did y'all build that in my neighborhood?" We were telling him about it and he was like, "Ooo, I don't want that shit in my neighborhood!" and he came back up the streets and he was like, "Hey, I got some CDs—y'all wanna buy some?" And then he was like, "I gotta sister, man. I gotta sister. She fixin' to get out, can y'all help my sister?" I was just like, see, look at God. Look at God. That's what it is. It's a light. And we light our candles—that's what we say at the beginning of just about every group that we have: "We light the candle for the women that have lost their way to be able to find their way back, and for the women who don't know this way of life, that they'll see the light—the flame—and they'll come towards it." And we say that we are the flame. We're the candle. We're the light. That's what I tell the women in the program now, all the time: be careful when you walk out of these doors, because you would be surprised who's watchin' you—you're an ambassador, you're a representative of Magdalene. Magdalene is you—the gift that's been given to you. You know what I'm saying? So if you are grateful for the gift, then carry yourself like the gift. A grateful addict will never use again. I know that to be true in my own life. If I'm really practicing some gratitude, I'm not tempted to use again. If I'm just following the way—I mean, nobody's perfect, I damn sure ain't perfect, but if I'm doing my best—if you're doing your best—we'll meet the mark. Just remember who you are and what you're doing.

How I ended up working for Magdalene: I finished the program in '99 and I was doing home health care, and I moved into my own home and got my children back, but I would still come over to the Magdalene houses. We had three houses at that time: the Park Avenue, the Arthur, and the Hillside. I would go to those houses and see if any of the women wanted to go to a meeting, or just check on 'em, you know. One of the greatest gifts that I got coming into Magdalene was that I had my own key, and I didn't have anybody there beating me over the head saying, "You gotta be here at 10:00, or 10:01," or "You're late," or "You're going to get kicked out," or whatever. There was no one making sure I got up, or making me get up out the bed, or do my chores right then, all that kind of stuff. I was being trusted to do the right thing even when nobody was looking. Magdalene trusted me to have a key to their house—they're not even here, but they're paying the rent, and all they want me to do is the right thing. We had a few rules, so we just had to follow the rules. That was a big deal to me—that somebody was trusting me with their environment: to take good care of it, and to do the right thing. So after I moved out, I would come back just to make sure that everybody's "doing the right thing." [*laughs*] Because I love this program, I became really protective of it. I didn't want anybody misusing the gift. So one day Becca asked me about my night job with the lady that I was sitting with, and then, she was just like, "Well, how much do you make there?" I told her and she said, "Well, what if I paid you to do what you're already doing? You come and check on the women all the time anyway. . . . If I paid you what they pay you, would you be willing to just come and be like the residence manager?" We didn't have a residence manager, so I asked, "So, we're going to start like having people live in?" And she was like, "No, you can live at home and just check on the houses, which you're doing." And I was just like, "Well, hell yeah."

When I was in jail, I asked God that when I got out, if I could have a job where I could work with women just like myself. And, years later, that's what happened. Becca offered me this job as residence manager, which means that I check on the houses, take the women to meetings, make sure that they have all the house supplies, create retreats for us to go on—you know, for sisterhood and bonding—do peer counseling—it's a lot, you know. It's developed into a lot more, and it's brought me a lot closer to the women, and it's brought the women closer, too, because we get to go do different things together. That's a gift in itself, seeing the women come in like I was, curious and thinking, "What's the hook?" and "These people are crazy, they're not fixin' to just pay my rent," and "They have to be expecting something." Every single one of them comes in expecting somebody is wanting something from them. It's gotten better through the years, though, because our name is out there and the women have come through the program and they've talked about what a good program this is and how these people stick with us. It's not a federal agency or a government agency or a state agency or anything, but it's truly a gift from God—a gift from Becca and all the people that support Becca, that support us. The monies come in from supporters in the community—the community *does* care when we thought that they didn't. I've got the best job in the world, girl. It's stressful at times because I get to run into myself. I tell the women that they're mirrors for me. 'Cause I remember when I was rough. Well, I can still be rough. [*laughs*] And I remember when I was in disbelief and I didn't know if it was gonna work, and I remember acting out and being on plans and contracts, and I remember breaking rules and getting consequences and all of this stuff, and really just being determined to see, "Does this lady—is she for real? Is this program for real? Do they care?" At the beginning, I didn't know how to receive love, but I learned—am learning—how to. But the women are—they're mirrors of me at the beginning. It doesn't take long and I get to see them soften. Our symbol is the thistle, with the rough edges and the flower, and that's how we are, you know?

That's how we come in—we be rough, we got that street mentality, you know: "Ain't nobody gonna fuck with me" and "Get
out of my face" and whatever. And then the walls come down.
Watching the women be able to melt away all the stuff that happened back then and step into what can happen and what's possible now. Just watching their process is a gift in itself. So pretty
much what I do is encourage, inspire, motivate, I think. Argue.
[*laughs*] I have to show that rough side sometimes. "Go back
to the streets," that's what I say. "So we goin' back to the streets,
huh? Is that what we gotta do?" But we're all—it's a family. It's
a family. And in all families there's some kind of chaos and dis-
sension, but the thing of it is watching it, being able to com-
municate and work through it and watching the love come to
the surface again. Some days, some of the women living here
now be like, "I can't stand you!" [*laughs*] And it's like, "It's OK,
you'll love me again." I had one girl tell me—she was so mad
at me—and I was like, "That's OK, you'll love me again tomorrow." And she was like, "I don't love you! I'm not gonna love
you. I can't stand your ass." [*laughs*] And about three days later
she was like, "Marion, I love you." And I was like, "I love you,
too." I think back to her 'cause these women give me hell, and
there's twenty-two of 'em—twenty-two different personalities.
And, God, on most days, let's just say I have to practice the spiritual principles from the program that I'm taught, because on
any given day, man, it can be one or it can be all of them, trip-
pin'. In spite of it all, I *love* my job.

When I think back on my life, I thank God that Magdalene
was there for me. I was able to get some help for my addiction—my substance abuse, I was able to go to college, and I
was able to gain custody back of my children. I've been able to
hold down a legal job for thirteen years. I haven't had to sell my
ass, I haven't had to sell any crap to anybody to get high. The
number one precious gift in my life was being able to get my
sons back and be a mother to them. Because just leaving them,
and not wanting to—when you're on the drugs, people think
that you're choosing the drugs over your family, but that's not

the way it is. It's like you're so consumed, and I really believed the lie—I really believed that I could stop. But I couldn't stop without help, and then what I found out was that there was no help. Before Magdalene, there was nothing for the girls. There was nothing for women that wanted to turn their lives around— at least, nothing that I knew of. But when God gave this vision to Becca, it was a lifeline. Not just to me, but to women who truly wanted to get out but didn't know how to get out. This program centers around the specific issue of prostitution and there was nothing that addressed that. Nothing where we could have somebody really wanting to listen to us and care about us and care about the rapes, or how we got introduced to the streets, or why we sold ourselves, why we even thought that we had to have the drug, or even what happened before the streets. Like at home, you know, I have an uncle, and cousins that I was molested by, and the environment at Magdalene was safe and someplace where I could share all of that. We were all there and we all related and we were all connected in that way, because it just didn't happen to me, it happened to my sisters, too. Magdalene was a place where we could talk about it, and we had someone to encourage us to deal with those issues, and someone let us know that we could be better. We could walk better. We could do something totally different with our lives, whatever that may be. Becca just said, you know, "Whatever you want to do, I'm going to walk with you." And she did. Just to talk about it helps the healing—the slow process of healing—come on about much faster. There will be a process of healing—probably until I leave this earth, you know, because of everything that happened to me. But, I got my boys back. I got my boys back. For ten years, they were in my home with me. And here I am today, thirteen years later.

CHAPTER 4

Health and Healing

Seeking Definition

> Being healthy means I don't have to be on the streets
> today, and I am glad of that. Today, I can see light. I
> can get up. I can bathe. I'm in my right mind. I can ask
> for help, just a little. It takes courage to ask for help, for
> me. Every day I wake up and have breath, and I can say,
> "Thank you, God," that's a good day for me.
> —Gina, Magdalene House graduate

WHEN I ASKED WOMEN at Magdalene House what it meant
to be "well," they often started by telling me about what wellness is not. Their sense of themselves while they were on the streets—
and often after they had come off—was that they had a long way to
go in the journey toward healing. Their affection for drugs and alcohol had left them with damaged bodies, foggy minds, and broken relationships, and the mechanisms of survival on the streets had done
the same. Women described life on the streets as a constant cycle of
"rippin' and runnin'"—turning a trick to get money to get dope, getting
high to erase the memory of the trick, then tricking again to get more
dope, all the while walking the streets for days at a time without eating,
sleeping, or bathing. Kristen, a young woman who had dropped out of
college to use and to prostitute, told me:

I was really, really sick when I got to Magdalene. I had pneumonia,
I had just come off the streets, I was having seizures at the end of my
using. I didn't have any money, and my mom and dad had sent me
money but they didn't know where to send it to. I was so miserable
sick. I was really beat up from the streets. I couldn't hardly walk, my
feet were so blistered and bruised and my whole body—I mean, my
teeth were so messed up . . . my hair was coming out. I was really just
messed up when I got here.

In addition to illnesses caused by the hard life of the streets, many
women had or developed illnesses that went untreated during their addiction. Shelly described using drugs to "treat" her diabetes, saying:

I didn't think about it, I guess. I didn't have my medication, so I knew I
was sick, you know, but I just—I was using drugs, and really I felt that's
what my medication was, opposed to my insulin, you know what I
mean? And several times I wound up in the emergency room because
I would not take my insulin or my pills, or my blood pressure would
rise and I wouldn't take that medication. I thought as long as I was
gettin' high, that was it, you know?

Sherri, who discovered she had breast cancer shortly after she entered
the Magdalene program said, "If I hadn't of been in the program, what
are the chances that I would have found out that I had the cancer? If I
had been out there using, there is no way I would have been going to
the doctor, you know what I mean, and taking care of myself. I think I
would have died from the cancer before I ever even knew I had it." Instead, she was able to get treatment for it, and she was surrounded by a
community of people who sat by her bedside when she was undergoing
chemotherapy, took her wig shopping when she lost her hair, and celebrated with her when the cancer was deemed in remission.

The women also talked about what it meant to be mentally "un-
well." For most of them, depression was the marker of poor mental
health. Kayla said:

When we first come in from the streets—well, when many of us
first come in from the streets, we suffer from post-traumatic stress
syndrome. Same thing that men in the war experience, and what I
think about is being violated at an early age—at age eleven—and how
I carried that for years. It was like a big domino effect—it affected all
areas of life. It made it easy for the drugs to just take hold. When I got
to Magdalene, I was depressed, you know? I was in a place of total
depression—I couldn't see anything positive, nothing was good. I
didn't have any hope—any reason to *keep* going other than that I was
too scared to *stop* going.

In one of the meeting rooms at Lena House, there is a photo-
graph of a woman with a small teardrop tattooed below her right eye. I
know that the woman used to be a resident, but I have never met her,
nor do I know her story. Perhaps she came through the program, got
clean, and moved on. Maybe she came off the streets for a while, relapsed, and went back. I often stared at her picture during meetings,
wondering about who she is. I wonder when, where, and why she got
her teardrop tattoo, particularly because most of the women I know at
Magdalene have enough outward, physical scars to make such a symbol unnecessary. Kayla has a scar where her neck meets her collarbone,
marking the place she was stabbed by a trick. The skin on Marion's
face is discolored from a burn she incurred when the "stove" on
which she was cooking her crack cocaine exploded. Toni never wears
shorts because she feels her legs are ugly from the abuse she sustained
at the hands of a pimp. Shadows of what were once bullet wounds,
knife marks, compound fractures, and other serious injuries grace the
flesh of the women who have known the violence of life in the mar-
gins. This makes me think that the teardrop must represent something
deeper than physical wounds. Something more persistent. Something
with a different kind of shadow. Reflecting on her battle with depression, Kayla said, "I can't imagine being in that place all the time. That
would be just as bad to me as being on the streets."

Depression often remains an ongoing struggle for women long after they arrive at Magdalene, as it is for approximately one in fourteen

Americans (Wang et al. 2005). Donna had been in the program for almost two years when she described a recent episode:

> I was not really talking. Just isolatin'. And I had done that for a
> couple of months. So, that's unhealthy for me: not reaching out,
> or telling somebody what's going on, or telling somebody how I'm
> really feeling, or whatever it is that could be going on—not doing
> that and just staying stuck. And I was staying stuck for a while. No
> groups, no meetin's. Wasn't talkin' to nobody and they would come
> to my room and I would just look at 'em like, "OK, you need to get
> out." But they wouldn't have it that way. And it took me a minute to
> really snap back, but I snapped back. And I'm still here, so. . . . It's
> been a journey.

For women such as Donna, the presence of faithful and persistent others was essential to the process of healing, and caring relationships with others were a marker of health. It is not surprising, then, that most women said that lost relationships were the signals that ultimately alerted them to the severity of their addiction—to how sick they really were. For Sandra, the loss was figurative:

> When I finally gave up and got help, it was because my granny
> had sent me my baby pictures, and—well, let me back up: When I
> was about six years old, I had said, "Grandmommy, when you die,
> can I have these pictures?" And I kept bugging her to send 'em to
> me, because I wanted to put 'em in a locket and send 'em back to
> her, so she finally sended 'em to me. I got out of jail, and the week
> after I got out of jail, someone stole all my stuff. He said, "You got
> some money?" I said, "No," but he just took my bag and took off
> walking. I couldn't find him or my pictures nowhere. I flagged down
> my friend and said, "Hey! Help me find this dude—he took all my
> stuff!" and we drove everywhere—we went in the truck stop, in the
> restaurant, but he was just gone. And . . . I was like, "Man, I can't
> take no more of this."

Sandra told me that losing her grandmother's pictures—her one record of life with her family—symbolized how deeply her addiction had affected her relationships with people she loved. Drug use and street life had helped her escape the people in her childhood who had harmed her, but her search for freedom and safety had also left her without those who loved and cared for her. Sandra was frightened by her own isolation and appalled at the cruelty of someone who would steal her pictures: "Not money. Not drugs. Not food, even. Pictures. *My pictures.*"

Other women lost loved ones to death and disease without being present to care for them, grieve, or say goodbye. They lost their children to state custody or more stable family members. These losses were often what brought women off the streets, but the journey was sometimes painfully long.

Choices

At Thistle Farms, I spent many hours in the office working with Natalie. We were companions during tedious but necessary tasks such as stuffing envelopes, running credit cards, and organizing supplies. I loved my conversations with Natalie—she was a disarming combination of gentle and frank, yet fiercely sarcastic. I learned much about the aftermath of addiction from listening to her describe her attempts to regain custody of her son, who was living with her parents. She had "dotted every i and crossed every t" in terms of what the courts had asked her to do: she had completed two years at Magdalene, she was participating in recovery meetings, and she had attended anger management classes, parenting classes, and therapy sessions. She had been cleared by her doctor as physically healthy and mentally stable. She had a job and a place to live. All these efforts, in her eyes, were evidence of how badly she wanted to be the person who cared for her son. "You want to know the really sick thing?" she asked me. "The really sick thing is that I remember when I was using and they took him, I was sad because he was gone, but I was also kind of happy because it meant that I could use more and not have to worry about him."

I became friends with Lucy, a volunteer at Magdalene whose daughter had fought a long battle with addiction. My friend found a great degree of comfort and community through Al-Anon, a twelve-step group for persons affected by their loved ones' struggles with substance abuse. Lucy said that participating in the group had been a healing experience for her, in particular because it had helped her make sense of what was happening in her own life as a result of her daughter's condition. She had learned that "if you're in a relationship with someone in active addiction, the thing you have to be OK with is that, at best, you'll always be number two. For people in active addiction, their substance of choice is their primary relationship."

Many of the women I interviewed described the effects of addiction in much the same way. Linda shared her own experience of choosing drugs over things that she felt should have been more important:

> There are things that I think about, like, "I missed seventeen years of my son's life," you know? Him just living a couple miles from me, and yet, I was lucky if I saw him two or three times a year. He just lived two miles from me. And *years* went by, you know? And I'm just now getting to really know my son. Five years ago, I couldn't tell you what his favorite color was, what his favorite movies were, what his favorite music was, what he liked to wear—I mean, you know, that's something that a parent just knows. When my son became old enough to put his foot down, he, you know, would say to me, "You have to make a choice, me or drugs." And I'd say to him, "Well, of course you're my choice," and "I'm going to stop." So if I thought I was going to see him, I would stop using for a day or two. In my mind, I thought I could trick him into believing I wasn't using, but you can't just go a few hours or a day and not use, with the intention of using again, because my whole everything was still all about the next time I was going to use. My reactions, how I spoke—you know, just *everything*. So . . . for years, he wouldn't really have anything to do with me. And it just didn't matter, really. It didn't matter. Not that I was saying, "Well, screw my son." It was like, I just thought, "Well, he's doing his thing, and I'm doing my thing." You know, but

. . . as I got older, I'm like, "Oh my God. I don't know who any of
my son's friends are, I don't know what he's doing with his life."

Linda's regret grew out of a sense that she had valued the wrong
things—that she had made poor choices. Whether or not prioritizing
illicit substances over personal relationships is any better or worse than
prioritizing more socially acceptable activities such as the pursuit of
wealth, power, or positive self-image is a worthwhile discussion that has
been taken up elsewhere (May 2007). For the purposes of understanding the women at Magdalene, however, it is important to understand
that their drug use went from being something that was recreational to
something that was all consuming and had dire consequences. Gayle
shared how it had consumed her:

> It started with just being a way for me to, like, relax, and I wasn't
> . . . able to deal with life, and it was like a way to escape for me, you
> know what I'm saying? It was a way to escape—it was fun and it was
> like every weekend or every other weekend, and then it became
> during the weekdays and interfering with my job, and my kids, and
> being a mother, and stuff like that. When I decided I wanted to be
> a mother again, I found out that I had a problem and that it was
> affecting my kids, and my mom, and my friends—I had no social
> life. I had no idea what progression was, like with the disease and
> stuff, and it started to progress until I was addicted, and by the time
> I started to realize all that, my disease was full blown. And so at
> that point, I went straight from there to denial—that I didn't have a
> problem. Everybody saw that I had a problem but me, and I really
> didn't think that I was hurting nobody else. "It was my life," and "I
> ain't hurtin' nobody," you know, so, for me, that took place for like
> fourteen years.

For women at Magdalene, addiction had played a primary role in their
lives, and it had often become a defining characteristic of their self-
images. Sometimes they viewed it as a disease, at other times as the
result of difficult life experiences, and still other times as the result of
poor choices. Notably, the narratives that accompany addiction and re-

covery shape those experiences for those who encounter them. Recent works on the role of narrative in providing scripts for addiction and recovery have observed that the stories we tell about addiction are important in constructing alternative "non-addict" identities (Rafalovich 1999; McKeganey and McIntosh 2000), combating stigma (Kondrat and Teater 2009), and negotiating localized cultural politics that shape definitions and beliefs about individuals who experience addiction and mental illness (Prussing 2007).

At Magdalene, the stories that accompany addiction find their roots in the twelve-step tradition of recovery, which conceptualizes addiction as a disease of the whole person and requires its followers to participate in a community of other addicts working toward wellness. Twelve-step traditions have often been criticized for moralizing the process of addiction and recovery, particularly by persons who ascribe to more biological or social models of addiction. For women at Magdalene, however, twelve-step narratives married to strong social critique and theological underpinnings seem to provide a mechanism through which addiction can be understood as a complex relationship between biological, psychological, spiritual, and social factors.

Like most narratives, the narratives within the Magdalene community about the meanings of addiction are activated strategically (Polletta 2006) and motivated by a variety of factors. First and foremost, narratives serve the purpose of holding out the possibility for change. Specifically, they form explanations of addiction that preserve a positive and mutable sense of self; the idea that "the things I've done" are not equivalent to "who I am" is important to this. For example, one morning at meditation, Natalie responded to a text about thinking of addiction as a disease by saying: "I really liked that reading, because that's something I think about a lot. I wish my family understood that addiction is a disease—I think they think I'm just a bad person. That I used drugs because I don't have any self control, or don't care about myself and the people around me. I've learned that I'm not a bad person. I have a *problem*."

For Natalie, understanding addiction as a disease meant that there was some explanation for her perceived lack of ability to stop using even if and when she wanted to. Furthermore, equating addiction with disease had a promising correlate—the opportunity for a cure. Other women relied on narratives that located their propensity to use and find comfort in illicit drugs in other factors such as family environments or past abuse. Because these factors were things of the past, drug use could be too. Kathleen said:

> I was always around stuff that didn't mean me no good, and to get on this side and to have somebody to care about me? To actually show me that they care about me? That's some healing. And what it did, it allowed me to go to those deep places that I experienced in my life. To talk about the molestation, to talk about the death, and grief. Talk about the abandonment. Talk about me being left, then walking away, leaving my kids. And I was able to heal from the past. It let me know that I wasn't a bad person, I just made bad choices.

Unlike Natalie and Kathleen, Sherri was resistant to the idea that her drug use or addiction was caused by some other factor—internal or external. She said, "I had a lot of issues, okay? . . . But once I did a little more work on myself, and I took a little bit more responsibility, I realized I *chose* to do what I did, OK? I can't blame my mom anymore, you know what I mean? Because there's just too much help out there, and I chose not to get the help, so I *chose* to do that. And I don't want anybody judging me, but I don't want anybody feeling sorry for me neither."

I have yet to meet a woman in recovery at Magdalene who would deny her own role in her addiction or addictions. Furthermore, the amount of shame and guilt that women experience as a result of addiction is often itself debilitating. Indeed, an important step in healing from addiction is finding a way to relieve some of the shame that women say can "keep you sick." Most women at Magdalene work tremendously hard to follow a program of recovery, and attribute their ability to heal (at least in part) to their own efforts. Still, it is important to emphasize that the environments in which women at Magdalene developed and experienced their addictions worked to shape those experiences into ones that were profoundly detrimental. At some level, most women at Magdalene (like almost everyone I know) felt that they had made poor choices at some point in their lives. The thing about choices, however, is that the contexts in which they take place *matter* in important ways (Nussbaum 2000; Hirschmann 2003), and the consequences of such choices are different for different people (Zerai and Banks 2002). Furthermore, the contexts and consequences are often not random, but rather tend to align themselves with existing injustices (Singer 2008). For the women at Magdalene, the availability of hard drugs, their previous encounters with abuse, and the consequences for mostly poor, mostly African American women using crack cocaine and heroin meant that their life experiences, their disease, and the choices they made led to particularly devastating results.

Going to Prison, Coming Out Sicker

Every woman I interviewed had been in correctional facilities multiple times before she came to Magdalene, some more than others. Sandra told me with a sheepish grin, "I've been going to jail constantly in this town. I like have 350 arrests for prostitution alone. Who knows how many for drugs." Most women had been to jail fewer times than Sandra, but recidivism rates were high for them all. This revolving-door phenomenon exists at least in part because jails and prisons are used as alternatives to treating drug use (Singer 2008), and because time behind bars is likely to make a person sicker, poorer, and less connected to the social supports that are necessary to facilitate recovery (Golembeski and Fullilove 2008). Activists have accused US state and municipal governments of using jails and prisons as holding cells for persons with mental illness, and the statistics appear to corroborate these claims. The incidence of serious mental illnesses is up to four times higher in prison populations than the population at large (ibid.).

Although the conditions in prison were sometimes better than the conditions of the streets, prison was a place that helped women "dry out," but did little in the way of providing support and pathways for healing. Furthermore, when women were released from prison, the communities into which they were released frequently lacked the necessary resources, social support, and service integration to make the transitions successful. In addition to the fact that unsuccessful transition is likely to lead to recidivism, the lack of community assistance means that the transition from prison to community is itself a health risk. A 2007 study of inmates released from a Washington state prison found that during the two weeks following release, former inmates were almost thirteen times more likely to die than the general state population. During that time period, former inmates were 129 times more likely to die of a drug overdose. The other leading causes of death (all at rates substantially higher than those of the general population) were cardiovascular disease, suicide, and homicide. Although the risk of death for former inmates declines significantly after the first two weeks following release, a two-year follow-up study demonstrated that it was still 3.5 times that of the general population.

The stories the women tell of going in and out of correctional facilities provide some degree of explanation for these statistics. They go into prison sick and come out sicker. They are released at 12:01 a.m. on the day their sentence expires, which means they are frequently put back on the streets in the middle of the night. Although there is usually some transition counseling done through the correctional system, women often leave it without a job, a permanent place to live, or any connection to resources that could help them get healthy. Of the women I interviewed who had received treatment, many of them expressed frustration with programs that either ignored or were not capable of addressing issues of childhood loss and trauma, abuse, and mental illness, saying that these programs had helped them get clean but not recover. According to the Magdalene database, which contains data on all residents who entered the program after 1999, approximately 80 percent of Magdalene participants meet the clinical qualifications for a dual diagnosis of substance use disorder with comorbid mental illness at any given time. Few if any of the women had been receiving mental health treatment before or during their time on the streets, joining 4.8 million other American adults who have reported needing but not receiving treatment for mental health problems (SAMHSA 2006). Similarly, 146,000 adult Tennesseans have reported needing but not receiving services for drug addiction, and 316,000 adult Tennesseans have reported a treatment gap for alcohol dependency (ibid.). For the women at Magdalene, however, lack of prior treatment for addiction was often less the problem than efficacy of services received. They had gone through a continual cycle of addiction and rehabilitation (either through treatment centers or correctional facilities) before coming to Magdalene. Although the cycle continues for some of the women, Magdalene was the end of the road for many of them when it came to their active addictions.

Eating Every Day, Sleeping at Night

According to women at Magdalene, there are specific qualities of the community itself that make it a place where, unlike correctional or standard treatment facilities, healing becomes possible. The road to recovery has meant, first and foremost, having the time, safety, and resources to heal. Gayle described how her time at Magdalene allowed her to access necessary resources that otherwise would not have been available to her: "When I think about it, a lot of stuff that has helped me to heal, like the positive people in my life, the encouragement, the counseling, the treatment and stuff . . . everything was free. And if I hadn't had Magdalene as a program, that has so many different areas that they help you work on—if I had done that individually, I wouldn't have been able to do some of that stuff" because of the cost. Gayle said that it had been a blessing not to worry about the cost or the "easy stuff that you don't think about, like being able to get there, to appointments. . . . Transportation was important, and so, healing to me looks like *all* of that."

Gayle's account of what helped her heal invokes capability theory, which has been espoused by Martha Nussbaum (2000), Amartya Sen (1999), and others. According to capability theory, justice and freedom (and in this case, health) are made possible when individuals reside in contexts that support human development with an array of basic provisions. Although capability theorists differ on the precise content of these arrays, the provisions include things such as housing, health care, and the ability to move about safely. A key premise is that the basic provisions are the starting point for human development, not the ending place: health and shelter aren't goods that one attains, but rather basic guarantees offered to all members of the human family.

Kathleen said that the provision of resources not only brought about physical well-being but also helped her believe something important about herself: that she was lovable. She explained, "By helping me, they loved on me before I was willing to love on myself, and that was healing for me." Gayle spoke of the compassion bestowed on her—"knowin' this person's not able to afford or able to get what they need, but givin' it to 'em"—and of wanting to "get better so I can then, too, give back what they've given me." For Gayle and Kathleen, the provision of resources and loving relationships was necessary to healing because they are requirements of human flourishing. According to Magdalene residents, graduates, and staff, they are necessary for another reason: they support the long, arduous task of healing.

When the women talked about their understandings of physical health, they mentioned basic, practical qualities and strategies for maintaining healthy bodies. Many expressed wonder that their bodies had held up to the abuse they had been through. They also offered descriptions of health that illustrated how deprived they had been when they were on the streets. Several women said things along the lines of "I eat every day" and "I sleep at night." Other markers of physical health included visiting the doctor, taking vitamins and medications, trying to exercise, and making good choices about food. These options, of course, did not become suddenly available when women left the streets and stopped using. They were, as Gayle described above, part of the provision that Magdalene made possible. To say that women at Magdalene might not have otherwise been able to afford or to access healthy food or adequate shelter is not an overstatement. In 2006, the US Department of Agriculture issued a report saying that the minimum amount a nonpregnant woman between the ages of twelve and fifty could reasonably spend on groceries and still eat adequately and healthily is $33.30 a week. In addition to the fact that this figure does not include the cost of transportation to stores that sell healthy food, and assumes access to such food, it is also 50 percent more than the weekly allocation of food stamps to a single adult. Similarly, housing options are often cost prohibitive, even when they ostensibly exist to provide affordable housing. For example, many halfway house pro-grams in Nashville provide apartments that rent for $75–$125 a week. Considering that the vast majority of the women leave jail, prison, or the streets without a job and often have difficulty getting one because of current employment regulations, it is not difficult to see how eat-ing every day and sleeping at night (not to mention going to the doc-tor and taking medication) are health markers they do not take for granted.

Being More Than Their Diseases

Women at Magdalene typically practiced a twelve-step program of re-covery, received counseling and therapy, and had access to medica-tions to treat mental illness. Despite knowing the statistics about the physical and mental health of the women at Magdalene as a group, I rarely knew which particular illnesses a woman did or did not have unless she told me. In general, I didn't ask—it didn't seem natural as a part of normal daily conversation, and besides, part of what made Mag-dalene a place that brought about healing was that it was a place where people could be more than their diseases. Because of this, perhaps, I often forgot that many of the women had severe mental illnesses, re-membering only when someone would mention needing to take a medication I knew to be for schizophrenia or another psychotic disor-der. This quality of Magdalene illustrates how diseases that *could* mean institutionalization, isolation, and disability can be transformed when women have access to proper treatment and membership in a com-munity structured to welcome and accommodate human difference. Furthermore, because Magdalene subscribes to a vision of well-being in which the journey of healing is lifelong and includes us all, it means that one does not have to be fully well to live fully. When I asked Mar-jorie about mental health, she talked about the importance of having dreams and the support to make them come true. According to Marjo-rie, being mentally healthy means "you can go beyond the skies, you know? Explore, you know? And anything positive that you even think you might wanna do, or anything that you see somebody else doin' it and you go, 'Huh, I wish I could do that'—don't wish, do it. You know what I mean? Do it. Just put forth that effort and you know if you take one step, God will take two."

Healthy Relationships

The dreams that the women most wanted to come true allude to another sign of wellness: healthy relationships. The dreams the women talked about were dreams of forming healing relationships and helping other people. Whether this meant caring for family members who had supported them during their addiction, or encouraging other addicts to seek treatment, it seemed that the surest marker of health was the ability to participate fruitfully in the lives of others. For example, Shelly described her plans:

> My completion date is April 11, 2010, and I am moving out of the
> Magdalene program as we speak. I'm going back to Detroit to bring
> my mom here with me. And I think that's a real big step. . . . I look
> at it as helping my mom come up out of the chaos. My mom isn't
> an addict, but she's living in chaos because some of my siblings are.
> So I'm going to go get her, and bring her, and that's another part of
> the healing process, you know? My mother has always taken care of
> us—I'm talking about myself and my siblings—and my mother has
> Alzheimer's, and I feel it's time for me to take care of her. . . . I think
> that that's something that God has brought me out of addiction to do.
> So I'm kind of happy with that, you know, because I miss her. Well,
> I miss all my brothers and sisters, and I've even asked my younger
> brother to come here and try to get his self together, but the choice is
> his, and whenever he's ready, I'll be here to help him.

As one might imagine, reestablishing relationships after long histories of addiction can be difficult. Often, these relationships require their own processes of healing, and depend on the kindness of friends and family members who have waited patiently and faithfully for change. Describing such a relationship, Kayla said:

I think I was blessed that my mom has always been a huge support to me, through my addiction, through my finding out that I was HIV positive, the prostituting—her knowing all of that, she has always just been a support person for me, and that kind of transferred over into my daughter. You know, she never told my daughter that I didn't love her. She always told my daughter, "Your mom loves you, she's just sick." So that's what she was raised with.

Kayla was aware that her daughter "has experienced some anger and all of that, but just the fact that I'm in her life today, and that I am achieving and blossoming, and blooming and growing, it has taken away some of that anger and pain that she feels. All she wants is for her mom to be there. So that is huge for me. This whole process would be much, much harder if I didn't have that support."

Freedom

When the women described healing and health in general, they often talked about their experiences in terms of freedom as opposed to wellness. Lack of freedom was equated both with experiences of incarceration and the bondage of addiction, whereas freedom implied being free from substance abuse and the oppression of life on the streets. For example, Linda told me, "I think you can be in a prison without being in a prison—without being in a physical prison, and that's what I was. I was in my own prison. Isolation, and, you know, just living a lie. Freedom to me today is being able to get up every day and do things with no guilt. I am who I am today, and I'm proud of who I am today. And I'm proud of where I came from."

Among the many phrases common to Magdalene culture is the claim that "freedom starts with healing." It appears on Thistle Farms materials, and women in the community often refer to the importance of "being free"—being free from drugs, free from the streets, free from men who abused them, free to imagine the lives they want to live, and free to pursue such lives. Although Becca once told me, "'Freedom starts with healing'—I don't know what that means, exactly," she then went on to say:

> Where freedom comes from and where it begins, I don't know, but freedom to me means freedom to make your own choices in the world—freedom to live how you want to live. Freedom from drugs, freedom from having to buy and sell your body, freedom from verbal or emotional abuse from *anybody*—you're free to walk away from it. Free to walk toward whatever you want to walk toward. I think that includes, you know, freedom from oppression by authority—whether it's judicial authority or church authority or whatever—that hasn't served you well. You're free to walk away from that. But also freedom to *be*. To be who you are. Who you were created to be.

The idea of freedom resonates with many in the community, and true to the spirit of the phrase, experiencing freedom has much to do with healing. Describing her definition of freedom, Demetria told me, "I ain't miserable no more. That's freedom. I don't have to say yes no more when I want to say no." For every resident at Magdalene, freedom had at least something to do with sobriety. Illustrating a common response to my question, "Talk to me about freedom," Katie replied, "Free to make a choice. . . . When you're using, you don't have a choice. It's all about using. You take the first hit, and that's all your mind thinks is more more more more more." Similarly, Shelly said:

> Freedom. Freedom from active addiction, and all the things that I have done to get some drugs. I don't have to do none of that again. That's a whole lot of freedom. And, sometimes, girl, freedom from me. [*laughs*] Because I'm a mess. When I went home for Christmas, I saw freedom in my mother's eyes when she looked at me. The freedom to say, "Oooh, my daughter looks beautiful." 'Cause my mother used to say, "You look like a racehorse," you know. I was like ninety pounds wet. But freedom to me is just the fact that I wake up, God wakes me up. God wakes me every morning. I can get out the bed. I can take my medicine. I can eat. I can drink coffee. And I can prepare myself for a productive day. That's freedom for me.

Traditional political theorists have understood "freedom" as a decid-edly individualistic concept regarding independent agents attempt-ing to act, to prevent others from acting, or to enable them to act. These theories are typically rooted in the philosophies of men such as Thomas Hobbes, John Locke, Jean-Jacques Rousseau, and John Stuart Mill, and draw on Isaiah Berlin's distinction between negative freedom and positive freedom. According to this distinction, negative liberty refers to an absence of external restraints that come from outside the self and are alien to the self. Negative freedom involves things such as not being interfered with by others, and it is defined in opposition to concepts such as obligation and authority (Berlin 1971; Hirschmann 2003). Positive liberty is distinct from negative liberty in at least three ways: (1) it is concerned with the conditions necessary to exercise in-dividual choice, (2) it involves a more contextual and communal no-tion of the self, and (3) it takes into account "internal barriers" such as uncertainties, fears, addictions, and compulsions that might interfere with the subject's "true desires" (Hirschmann 2003). More recently, theorists have demonstrated how difficult (and dangerous) it is to parse freedom in this manner, and have sought a more integrated perspec-tive that speaks to the ability of internal human factors to shape and be shaped by external human environments. Specifically, feminist theorist Nancy Hirschmann claims that separating these two concepts ignores the important relationship between external and internal barriers to choice and takes for granted the choosing subject as an independent agent. In response to this dilemma, Hirschmann proposes a definition of "freedom" that integrates the two:

> Freedom . . . is centrally about choice, a claim with which many
> mainstream freedom theories would agree. But choice is constituted
> by a complex relationship between "internal" factors of will and
> desire—impacting on the preferences and desires one has and how
> one makes choices—and factors "outside" the self that may inhibit or
> enhance one's ability to pursue one's preferences, including the kind
> and number of choices available, the obstacles to making the preferred
> choice, and the variable power that different people have to make
> choices. (ix)

Such a notion of freedom allows for considering the multiple forces that shape choice in a manner more acquainted with contexts and institutions as agents that can restrain or support freedom. Likewise, this conception pays more attention to the ways in which informal regulations such as norms, beliefs, relationships, and cultural expectations limit available choices and an individual's ability to make them.

The idea that freedom can be and is restricted by internal and external factors that are ultimately so connected that they work to constitute each other is reminiscent of similar ideas contained in theories about direct and structural violence. In this sense, the claim that freedom starts with healing—that being able to make choices and exercise one's will requires some degree of treatment for addiction, mental illness, and physical maladies—seems also to require its opposite—healing starts with freedom. For many of the women at Magdalene, the cycle of living on the streets, then prison, then back on the streets again meant that they spent most of their adult lives oscillating between an environment in which there were no restrictions and one in which there were only restrictions. By any description, both places were marked by scarcity and severe limitations on freedom. Illustrating how the complete lack of restrictions could (ironically) lead to lack of freedom, a Magdalene staff member said:

> I guess there's a difference between freedom and license, and the chaos that's bred by total lack of structure or obligation—what you might think of as "total freedom"—works against freedom in a sense. So, for example, when you're on the streets, there's no time shift. There's no time to get up, there's no alarm clocks on the streets, you just get up whenever. However, you're also sleeping in a crack house and your dealer or somebody else might come in and wake you up when you're passed out by slamming a two-by-four against your head and tell you to get back out on the streets.

Based on my observations and conversations at Magdalene, the type of freedom that provides the impetus for healing is freedom that is supported by clear and reasonable guidelines that are enforced and agreed on by the community itself. Lynn went on to say that the structure of Magdalene works to counteract what are often lifelong experiences of disorganization, chaos, and license that were mistaken for freedom. Explaining the connections, she said:

> For me, I have to go back and think about each individual woman's early experiences, and then throughout the course of their life, what their experience of authority has been, and typically, it has not been good. It has not been nurturing, it's not been healthy for them. It's not been life enhancing, it's not been positive. And so . . . I would hope the gift of Magdalene would be to give somebody a respite in life to heal. You know, the best we can offer—the best we can aspire to every day—is to be a benevolent enough community that people get the time, the resources, and the relationships they need to be well.

Health, God, and the Loving Community

Miss Gina was Magdalene's oldest resident, and the resident with the poorest physical health, at least in any observable sense. Gina had chronic obstructive pulmonary disease (COPD), a progressive illness she had developed after "too many years of hittin' the pipe." As a result of her COPD, Gina was constantly out of breath, and at times her wheezing was so bad that I thought she might stop breathing altogether. Every few months or so, Gina felt bad enough that Holli would send someone from Thistle Farms to take her to the hospital.

Holli called the ambulance for Gina twice. Early in the spring of 2008, I showed up at Thistle Farms one sunny Monday morning to learn that Gina had entered the hospital over the weekend with pneumonia, and no one expected her to live more than a few days. Magdalene residents, graduates, staff, and volunteers kept a constant vigil at the hospital—keeping Gina company, praying for her, and preparing her for death. Gina was stuffed full of tubes and attached to too many machines to count. The beeps drowned out her wheezing. She floated in and out of consciousness as everyone else waited. And waited. And waited. A few days after she should have been dead, Gina turned a corner and her pneumonia went away. Two weeks later, she rumbled up to Thistle Farms in her old beat-up car, walked up the path, and, in between wheezes, said with a shrug, "I guess God wasn't done with me yet."

Gina almost died two more times while I was working at Magdalene, and each time it was the same—community members would gather in the hospital, everyone (including Gina) would be certain that death was imminent, and then as quickly as she got sick, Gina would bounce back, always with the same response: "I guess God's not done with me." Sometimes I wondered if she wished that God would either be done with her or heal her COPD, but as far as I could tell, no one else considered that a possibility, so I didn't bring it up with her. Gina understood illness to be her path to community, relationships, and most importantly, to God. She saw her illness as a tool that helped her understand the sickness and suffering of others, and every "healing" as an opportunity to experience God's mercy and grace, which, she often reminded us, "are new every morning." Her understanding of health encompassed something broader than proper physical functioning—it involved a belief that her weakening body was making room for a stronger soul, and that her experience of health was deeply intertwined with participation in a loving community.

CHAPTER 5

St. Benedict's Ghost

Hospitality as Community Practice

> Recovery has to start with the kind of welcoming
> hospitality that has no conditions—full of healing, full
> of learning, and full of love.
> —Thomas, Magdalene House board member

AS DESCRIBED BY THE women of Magdalene House, the streets
are a conundrum of paradoxes: time is at once nonexistent and
pressing, space is always present but never available, and resources
are painfully close but desperately out of reach. On the one hand,
there is no measure or restriction of time—nowhere to be, no one to
meet, and no responsibilities to uphold. The women spoke of going
for months at a time without knowing what hour the clock showed,
what day the calendar read, or how long it had been since they last ate,
bathed, or slept. The only event that marked the day with meaning or
structure was the possibility of turning another trick to get one more
hit. At the same time, the fight for survival meant that the pace of life
on the streets was frenetic. Kayla said, "The chaos of the streets makes
you focus only on surviving. You don't have time to assess your situation, and you don't have time to even plan beyond right now—you're
just surviving." And this, she added, makes it difficult to envision other
ways of being: "You can't deal with your past or even worry about your
future. You can't do anything but face your present situation because
it's so chaotic." Likewise with physical space: women at Magdalene

had walked alone, night and day, through parts of Nashville that most people would be too scared to traverse. They had lived in abandoned houses, motel rooms, and under bridges. The freedom to move about was unrestricted; the ability of finding a new place to crash was always a possibility. At the same time, the houses in which they lived had been raided often, the motel rooms evacuated, and the bridges flooded. The women had been frequently exposed but rarely visible, at least to the gaze of most of Nashville's inhabitants. Having a physical (not to mention emotional) space that was reliably available, safe, and private was a privilege few women at Magdalene had enjoyed.

Healing, then, required more than personal commitment, loving relationships, and access to treatment. It required an environment—a community—in which the values that serve to govern daily life could be disciplined and reordered. "According to what?" is a fair and obvious question, although the answers imply that the more appropriate query would be "According to whom?" Describing her resistance to running a program that would have to answer to authorities outside the community, Becca Stevens said, "I didn't want to do any government stuff because I hate government stuff. And I didn't want to do a church thing because I hate church things. I just wanted it to be really easy for the women—just, you come in, relax, and we'll figure it out."

"Figuring it out" is an approach that has allowed the community to grow and evolve, all the while acknowledging the larger, unanswered questions implicated in the quest for healing. The persons whose beliefs and commitments structure the Magdalene community are many, and for this reason, perhaps, the standards by which the community is ordered are broad in scope and simple in definition: the community and those within it are shaped by practices of hospitality rooted in gratitude.

Magdalene's commitment to hospitality grows directly out of its affiliation with Benedictine theology. The Rule of St. Benedict, written around 500 CE, is a guide for living in monastic community. Many of its seventy-three chapters outline practices and disciplines that are not observed or emphasized in the Magdalene community, such as observing the Daily Office, agreeing to communal ownership of material possessions, and practicing moderation in eating, drinking, and speech. Indeed, my experience at Magdalene taught me that eating, talking, laughing, and arguing occur in abundance, while the twelve-step commitment to total sobriety means drinking has no place at all. Other Benedictine beliefs and practices, however, are clearly reflected in the daily gathering to read and meditate, the centrality of community, and the emphasis on hospitality. Hospitality, according the Benedictines, means that everyone who comes to the monastery—the traveler, the poor, the curious, and those of different religion, social status, or educational background—should be received with genuine acceptance and reverence (de Waal 2001). The reverence comes from the Christian understanding that in receiving strangers, one is receiving Christ himself. Hospitality, then, means welcoming in, sharing with, and providing for those who would never be expected to reciprocate. In this sense, it is regarded one of the "great sacrifices" of community (de Waal 2001)

At Magdalene, hospitality means that women are welcomed off the streets, treated with dignity, and offered resources to live, time to heal, and space to thrive. Women often say that the hospitality of the Magdalene community is what gave them the courage to start dreaming about a way of life other than what they had known on the streets. In *Find Your Way Home*, one woman recounts how she was living near Lena House when she started to get to know a few of the residents. The women at Lena frequently offered her food, clothing, and companionship. When this woman tells her story of recovery, she says, "It all started with a bag of chips," illustrating how small acts of compassion and inclusion wooed her toward healing community.

Hospitality as Provision of Resources

Like all wisdom at Magdalene, the guidance of St. Benedict is tempered, adapted, and understood through the lens of common experience. Talking about the importance of offering help and hospitality unconditionally, Becca described how this practice arose out of her own experience of growing up with little money. Becca's father died when she was six years old, and her mother was left to raise and provide for five children. Often, she said, obstacles that might have seemed trivial to someone with the resources to manage them would end up derailing an entire day:

> I know the stress of money in my background. For example, when I was growing up, a flat tire could ruin our whole day. Like, "we are not going to have enough money to fix the tire, then mom's not going to get to work, so we're going to have even less money, and it's going to be a roller coaster of problems." And I hated it. I hated the stress of that. And I didn't want people to turn a flat tire into a theology or a philosophy or a way to teach a lesson. Sometimes a flat tire is just a flat tire. As a kid, I would wish, "Just please give us fifty dollars, don't say anything, and keep going." That would have been the kindest thing that anyone could have done for us. Not give us a speech about how "you should have saved fifty dollars." Anyway, I know from my own experience that it's really difficult when you're struggling with no money, and I know the women coming out of jail or off the streets don't have any money, and so I wanted to just *erase* that.

Becca went on to describe specific ways that Magdalene works to alleviate the stress of money for the women who walk through its doors:

> I think it's oppressive to take people from jail into a halfway house, where they are required to pay $125 a week. If you have no work history, no jobs in your future, it is hard to come up with $125 a week for rent. And that's before anything else—before bus passes, before groceries, before paying court costs. You know, everything is so expensive when you have no transportation, and you're trying to get back and forth to work, and you have no clothes. I mean, there are legitimately so many things people need to live, and you're talking about women with *at best* sketchy job histories—some of them no job history, at least nothing legal. So [charging rent] never made any sense to me because all you're asking people to

do is go hustle or go sell drugs. And that's the thing that people say sometimes when they get desperate for money—they say, "I'm just gonna stay clean and sell the drugs. This time I'm not gonna use 'em." That's crazy. There's no way. So running a recovery program and charging people rent—I think it's oppressive, and I think it's cruel, and I think it's setting people up for failure.

Anyone who pays rent or a mortgage knows that the cost of safe, clean, and comfortable housing can be a burden. Imagine, then, trying to take on this burden with no job, a poor job history, and a criminal record that precludes you from qualifying for employment in all but a very few locations. Imagine further that the surest way to make the money you need to afford basic necessities is—for reasons of habit, skill, and social connections—to contact your dealer, pimp, or friends from the street. Imagine spending time in prison, getting clean, and being released into a world in which you are far more likely to be homeless than to be housed, to relapse than to stay clean, and to have myriad social, political, and economic factors driving you back to prison instead of trying to help you stay out (Golembeski and Fullilove 2005; Singer 2008). It is from these circumstances that women come to Magdalene, which promises them a place to live and heal—for free—for two years. Even among recovery programs, living space for free, and for that long, is rare. Katie said:

> I had tried other programs where, well, with most of them, you
> have to pay $100 a week in rent and I just, I was living there,
> following the rules, but there wasn't any love in the program. And
> I'm spending all this money on rent, but when my ninety days are
> up, what am I gonna do now? So I didn't have any hope or faith in
> those programs, so I just gave up and went back to the streets. And
> when I found out about Magdalene—it's a two-year program and it's
> rent free—I felt like that was time to really work on myself and save
> money and that way when the two years is up, I will have money,
> I'll be able to get a place and a car—everything that I need to live
> my life on my own. 'Cause I wanted to get off the drugs, but I didn't

want to depend on my family. Like, I didn't want my mom helping or anybody else. I just wanted to do it on my own. So I felt like Magdalene was a great opportunity to do that.

As described earlier, in addition to providing rent-free housing, Magdalene also gives each woman a weekly stipend during her first ninety days in residence. During that time, she is charged with a single job: to rest and to heal. Explaining the importance of these provisions in the healing process, Becca said:

> The stipend means that women are free from having to ask anybody for anything. They don't have to go to a man that has abused them in the past and ask him for fifty dollars for, whatever, cigarettes and bus passes and whatever a person needs to get through the week. So we provide the women with everything they need to live, so they're freer to focus on some of the real issues that you need to be dealing with, i.e., recovery. So those are the provisions we offer specifically, for the health of people.

Once women have begun to heal, they have the opportunity to work at Thistle Farms. Most women living in the Magdalene community work at the company at some point during their two-year stay. Some women work there briefly and then go on to other jobs, whereas some stay for longer. As of 2010, Magdalene residents and graduates filled all the full-time staff positions at Thistle Farms with the exception of the managing director and the chemist who develops and tests new products. This means that making lavender lotion was Toni's specialty; Glenda and Terri were the candle experts; Susan was in charge of labeling; Cindy trained new employees; Kayla, Deandra, and Bonnie served as sales representatives to stores carrying Thistle Farms products; and Minda managed the shipping department. It is the hope of the community that the managing director and chemist positions will also eventually be filled by Magdalene graduates. Additionally, the community's plan is for Thistle Farms to become big enough to provide challenging, full-time employment to women who want to make working at Thistle Farms their career. In the meantime, the company provides two to three years of employment for each woman at Magdalene who needs or wants to work at Thistle Farms. Beyond that, the company provides employment indefinitely for the women who would likely experience exclusion from other places of employment because of severe mental illness, learning disabilities, or extensive criminal records. Describing why it is important to provide employment for women such as Susan, who has not been able to obtain an outside position, Becca said:

> You're talking about a woman who cannot get hired at Goodwill. Goodwill will not hire Susan, or will not work with her for whatever reasons. And that does something to you, you know? Susan's sick, and she may never be completely well from some of the stuff she's dealing with, but because she gets money for coming into work, and being there at this company, I think that gives her a big gift of freedom and pride and all kinds of stuff.

According to the women at Thistle Farms, the importance of holding a job, showing up for work, and contributing to something about which one feels proud goes beyond financial provision. Corroborating a large body of scholarship, the women demonstrate that an important piece of maintaining mental health is having the opportunity to work (Fryer and Fagan 2003).

This is true for reasons other than economic stability, although being able to work to have money for basic needs is indeed important. Nearly every woman who comes to work at Thistle Farms talks about what a difference it is for her to get up in the morning and "do something good." I have seen a woman cry because she received her first paycheck in twenty-five years. I have seen a woman dance around the room the morning after an event because she had been entrusted with $900 in cash from product sales and managed to keep the money all night "without stealing a dime." While these may appear to be small wins (or perhaps even tokenistic involvement in the economic system), they were real and meaningful victories for the people who won them.

These stories represent the qualities that are deemed "good" in our society as well as reflecting what the women were excluded from while they were addicted, in prison, or on the streets.

Hospitality as Provision of Space and Time

In addition to providing housing, stipends, and employment, Magdalene also provides space and time, which are necessary to good health. The provision of housing is an obvious example of providing space, and residents, graduates, and staff say that the qualities of the space are part of what makes the environment conducive to healing. Living unsupervised in a safe, lovely, and loving home provides generative support to women as they heal. "Space" refers to more than just physical space, however. It also refers to the emotional and relational space Magdalene offers to its residents to allow them room to discover themselves. Describing the importance of this type of space, Kayla said:

> When you go to the regular treatment centers, there's like this across-the-board plan for everybody. Well, everybody's different. You know, we all come from different backgrounds; we were all raised differently. In Magdalene, each lady has her own individual plan, according to what her needs are. So that was different from the other treatment centers that I had been to. They sat down, and they looked at some of the things that I had been through in my life, how I was raised, and then they asked me, what was it in life that I wanted to do? And that was the first time anyone had ever taken the time and asked me what *I* wanted to do.

Giving women the opportunity to dream is a grace that many of them have rarely experienced. In addition to supporting the women's goals for big life decisions—career, family reunification, housing—Magdalene also works to make the "small things" work as well. For example, when Gayle began to heal, she told the program director that she had always wanted to know how to play the piano. Sonya communicated this information to Magdalene's volunteer coordinator, who then added "piano teacher for Gayle" to the list of needs included in each month's newsletter. A volunteer came forward to teach Gayle to play the piano. Gina decided she wanted to take art lessons, so Ruth, a volunteer at Thistle Farms, taught Gina how to paint. For the 2008 holiday season, Gina painted a white dove on a colorful background that served as the cover image for all of Magdalene's holiday cards. In the spring of 2009, Magdalene hosted an art auction for Gina and other community members who have begun to paint, draw, and create other forms of visual art. These and other provisions of space and time are a direct outgrowth of what members of the Magdalene community have learned it takes to heal.

The Process of Healing

The process of recovery is often understood to be a process of putting the pieces of self back together. For women who have experienced childhood abuse and trauma, long-term drug use, destitution, and violence done to their bodies and minds, illnesses such as dissociative disorder and post-traumatic stress disorder are common if not standard (Bolton et al. 2004; Christensen et al. 2005). In these disorders, the "self" scatters, enabling the individual to disengage mind from body in order to cope with the physical and psychological pain (Brison 2002; Morrison and Severino 2009). One of the first steps of healing as described by the women at Magdalene is the often-painful process of reintegration. During one of my group interviews, I asked the women who were participating what the process of healing looked like for them. Their responses:

> KAYLA: Well, for me, my process was pain, then love, and then revisiting the pain, then happiness. Because what I had to do in my therapy was I had to revisit the sexual abuse that happened to me at age eleven, and it was real painful. So I had to revisit that pain in order to get to a place of healing. I remember doing therapy [for] years, and they never discussed that. They only talked about what I wanted to talk about. This time, the therapist said, "We're going to visit some painful

places," and that's what healing was for me—revisiting pain in order to get to some freedom and some healing.

DONNA: Healing is like growing pains. It's like you have to go through something in order to grow from it. 'Cause it seems like it takes something horrible or dramatic to even make me pay attention to myself. And I hate that it's like that, but for me, that's what it takes—something to happen before I start trying to do something for myself. So once the healing process begins, it's kind of rough in the beginning. But as it goes on, it feels better. Knowing that what you're going through is to help you. And it's not just to help you, but it also helps the ones who're behind you, and your kids and the ones who're around you, so, it's real good. It feels real good.

KATHLEEN: All my life I felt pain. Coming up, you know, being a little girl that was talking out loud about being molested, but then my own mama and my own aunties wasn't hearing me. So I found myself doing things because he showed me love, but he really didn't love me, he would just buy me things so he could do it again. And when I came to Magdalene, and the pain started to go away, I thought something was wrong with me, because I had felt pain all my life. And it took my counselor to tell me there wasn't nothing wrong with me, I just didn't have to feel pain anymore. And it was scary because how do you just not feel pain anymore when that's all you've ever felt, you know? But I got through it and now I don't have to feel pain anymore to feel normal. I can laugh today. I can tell someone that I'm hurting today. I can actually tell myself I love *me* today when I couldn't love myself before, and I know that's healing.

SHERRI: Healing? What does it look like for me? In the beginning, it's very painful. In order to heal, you have to deal with the stuff that led you to the dope in the first place. And so the process of healing is rather difficult—there's nothing easy about it. Because you have to relive a lot of stuff, you know what I mean? And so, healing to me, in the beginning, is painful, and in the end, after you go through the process of it—I can't even think of words for it. It's just *life*, you know what I mean? It's a second chance, it's a family, it's—there's just so much that healing did for me. I have a relationship with my mom that I never thought I would have. I got two children that I didn't think I could have—I was told that I couldn't have children. I got married, I own my own home. So, I mean, healing kind of gave me life, if that makes sense. But it was a hard process. Sometimes I didn't want to do it—I felt like running. Sometimes it's easier to run than to deal with abandonment issues, sexual abuse issues, physical abuse issues, mental abuse issues, and I had all of that, you know? I didn't get stuck with just one or two—I had to get it all.

Although these descriptions were somewhat different from one another, common threads were present in each. Notably, all the women described healing as a painful process that requires difficult, continuous work and a strong, resilient community prepared to accompany and facilitate their healing. For these reasons, community members say that healing is a mysterious process that needs a hospitable community in which to unfold. In Becca's words:

It takes two years just to get strong enough to really deal with the issues. It's hard to imagine a person coming into a treatment or a recovery program who is dealing with deep, childhood, traumatic issues, and it taking *less than* two years. It takes a long time to even realize you're dealing with them. And then you just need everybody to be patient with you. And your body will sort it out and your mind will sort it out if there's a healing, safe community around you, and people obviously who are capable of dealing with that type of stuff.

Magdalene's approach to healing through hospitable provision of resources, space, and time is somewhat unusual in a world in which illnesses are increasingly treated by prescribing quick pharmaceutical solutions rather than addressing underlying causes. To be clear, access to necessary treatment (including pharmacological treatment) is essential to recovery for most women at Magdalene, and the community works diligently with physical and mental health providers in the Nashville area to make sure women have access to services. Science and modern medicine have, of course, made many important advances in technique; however, the sheer magnitude of illness and suffering in the world today begs the question of whether or not we might be missing something when it comes to healing.

The nineteenth-century philosopher Gabriel Marcel wrote that the result of living in a broken world is an increasingly detrimental desire to control the world through technical means. He claims that we experience the unknown as a problem to be solved by technical, impersonal means, as opposed to a mystery to be approached through participation and engagement. Practices such as breaking things into parts, quantifying them, and developing general theories with which to predict their likely behavior are examples of such technical attempts to understand and control the world (Marcel 1951). If, however, healing is a mysterious process, as the women at Magdalene say, it means that the process requires walking together, one step at a time, in a community that provides security along with solutions, and companionship in addition to cures.

Hospitality as Security of Membership

Early in my time at Magdalene, I learned that the residents were the central and primary members of the community. While this is not always true in terms of power structure or decision-making, it is true in terms of having a place of belonging in the Magdalene circle and having ownership of economic resources. For example, during a particularly bad economic season at Thistle Farms, Holli, the managing director, had the task of reducing spending. This could have been done any number of ways, of course, but the community was clear about how it would *not* be done: none of the Magdalene residents or graduates would lose their jobs, have their hours cut, or stop receiving food and gas stipends for work-related trips. Neither would Thistle Farms stop making and selling products. Rather, several part-time staff members were either let go or agreed to "volunteer" by working without pay. The staff members let go were those who could most afford it financially—virtually no other qualification was taken into consideration.

Although there were some hurt feelings, the general consensus was that this was the right decision—that Magdalene exists for the women coming off the streets, and continuing in this purpose required cutting the people who could most afford to go without the extra income. It is worth noting (and probably goes without saying) that this is not a typical hiring and firing practice. In an economic world where individual performance and efficiency are the grounds that merit employment, people would never be kept in a job because they are the least able to find another or afford to live without it. Magdalene works out of a different system, however—one in which providing for the women at the heart of the community is the ultimate bottom line.

The same is true when it comes to residency in the Magdalene houses and reliance on Magdalene resources. Although women are encouraged to move out of their rooms after they have completed their two years in the program (and most women are quite ready to leave by then), Magdalene has two transition houses to aid women as they establish independent housing, and I have known Magdalene to allow residents to stay in the recovery houses or the transition houses beyond the allotted time. Furthermore, Magdalene often continues to serve as a safety net for former residents after they move out and move on. It is not uncommon for a woman to lose her job and come back to Thistle Farms to work, or for women to turn to Magdalene in cases of an emergency. Twice during my time at Magdalene, former residents lost their homes when their apartment complexes caught fire. Both times, staff, volunteers, and graduates offered temporary housing, donated household items, and stepped in to provide emotional support.

Hospitality at Magdalene is extended to "strangers" as well. Every Wednesday morning at Thistle Farms, visitors and volunteers join the meditation circle to listen to stories and share their own. Some people come faithfully each week, others every once in a while, and still others come once and never return. People come because they've heard about the program, or because they have a friend who volunteers. They come because they're curious, seeking healing, in need of companionship, or eager for a new experience. In the two years I was at Thistle Farms, high school students, college students, journalists, musicians, photographers, business men and women, lawyers, doctors, church ladies, and neighbors all joined the circle. Whoever they were and for whatever reasons they had come, people were always welcome. This attitude is core to Magdalene and grows out of a belief that there is little to hide and plenty to share. The residents, staff, and volunteers at Magdalene say they have been given so much that there is no reason not to invite others into the community to experience the same gifts of friendship and healing.

Rooted in Gratitude

Although Magdalene works to provide women with safe and comfortable housing, financial security, health and education needs, and time to heal, with the conviction that these are basic necessities that *should* be offered to all human beings, the response of the women who receive them is far more often one of gratitude than entitlement. Robert Emmons (2007) defines gratitude as a practice of affirming goodness and recognizing that at least some of the sources of this goodness are outside the self. Residents at Magdalene are quick to name God, Becca, staff, volunteers, donors, graduates, and other residents as people who have helped them on their path to healing. Similarly, volunteers often express deep gratitude to residents and other members of the community for allowing them to take part in the work and the relationships that make Magdalene a place of love and healing. The acknowledgment of material and relational provision doesn't stop there, though; gratitude is part of the narrative that shapes and defines the Magdalene community as a whole. Expressing her gratefulness for the monetary provision that has allowed Magdalene to stay open, grow, and remain financially solvent for thirteen years, Becca remarked, "It just seems unbelievable that there's been so much given to this community: millions and millions and millions and millions of dollars have been given to this community. And it's all been given joyfully, pretty much. [*laughs*] And it's all been, hopefully, given back to the program and to the women, and then they give back to other people, and it just seems like such a surprise—so bountiful and so abundant."

For Magdalene in particular, gratitude represents an understanding of the world as a realm in which God is life-giving and generous, and people—all people—are dependent on the goodness of God and others for their lives and livelihood. Among other things, this belief generates a narrative that instructs residents, staff, and volunteers alike on the things they have being things they have been *given*, rather than things that they have earned.

It is important to recognize, however, that a theology of gratitude has the potential for abuse. One could imagine it going far astray if it was used to placate those who have experienced deep injustice or inequality (as most of the women at Magdalene have) by reminding them to be grateful regardless of circumstance, or similarly, that things could always be worse. Furthermore, gratitude has the potential to eclipse structures of injustice if it is understood in such a way that makes it seems as if the resources "we" have been "given" were given arbitrarily, rather than distributed along the lines of existing inequalities, which history (especially recent history) has taught us is most often the case (Farmer 2005; Sen 1999). At the same time, gratitude has the potential to be subversive because, in the words of Robert Emmons and Michael McCullough (2004), "We . . . do not like to think of ourselves as indebted. We would rather see our own fortunes as our own doing. . . . Like trust (to which it is closely akin), gratitude involves an admission of our vulnerability and our dependence on other people" (v).

In this sense, the claim that "everything is a gift" turns on its head what most of us think about deservingness through merit—if everything is a gift, it means that none of us "deserve" what we have, whether what we have is a bed at Magdalene or a large house in a nice neighborhood. Understood this way, gratitude is a narrative by which the many relationships, resources, and interdependencies necessary to support a life marked by flourishing are made visible. And visibility is especially important, say care theorists and theologians, in a world riddled with the myth of the self-made, autonomous individual who earns his or her flourishing through hard work and responsibility. According to these theorists, the myths mask and marginalize human need for each other (Tronto 1993; Kittay 2001), and for God and God's creation (McFague 2001; Wirzba 2006). From this perspective, gratitude can be used to create something of a different economy—an economy in which people with less are as deserving as those with more, and one in which admitting need can lead to power and companionship instead of poverty and isolation.

The Limits of Hospitality

Embracing practices of hospitality and gratitude can be difficult (if not in fact somewhat detrimental) when they conflict with the practices embraced by the social and economic context in which Magdalene resides. Learning how to practice them while protecting the integrity of the community requires balancing between extremes and accepting compromise on some issues. While St. Benedict emphasized hospitality in his rule, he also had careful guidelines governing the limits to welcoming strangers. In particular, he was concerned with "lingering guests," saying, "Too great a merging of monastics and guests will benefit neither" (de Waal 2001). Although Magdalene has little concern over the mingling of monastics and guests, and one could appropriately say that its approach to healing encourages guests to linger, there are limits to hospitality that exist for the purpose of maintaining the community.

First and foremost is the obvious limitation that a program that houses only twenty-two women must necessarily turn many women away. Although there are several other respectable recovery organizations and programs in Nashville from which women can receive treatment, Magdalene's waiting list demonstrates the large number of people who would like to be a part of the program but are not. Staff members report that different women call their offices every day, asking to get in, and there is often little that Magdalene personnel can do beyond referring the women to other services and programs. Magdalene's commitment to providing deep and lasting hospitality to each person in its program means that its reach is relatively narrow.

For women who do make it into the program, hospitality stops with behaviors or arrangements that the staff and other residents perceive to be detrimental to the healing process. Although the Magdalene program is known for having far fewer rules and regulations than many recovery communities, most people agree that at least some structure and restriction is necessary for the realization of healing. In addition to participating in the program activities described in Chapter 2, women must abstain from drugs and alcohol as long as they are living in Magdalene residences, and they are not allowed to have children or other family members live with them.[1] Aside from these requirements, there are a number of rules and expectations that govern behavior in the residences, including adherence to a midnight curfew, displaying respect for other people and their property, and completing household chores. Once a resident begins working at Thistle Farms, she is expected to show up for work consistently and on time, be responsible for her assigned tasks, and participate in continuing education opportunities. Ideally, the women in the community enforce these responsibilities themselves, but in reality, the authority of staff is often required as well. The idea that the restriction of some freedoms is necessary to the enjoyment of others is not new, nor is the idea that participation in any community requires varying degrees of conformity; however, the often-present conflict between freedom, restriction, and conformity is particularly salient at Magdalene. Lynn is a staff member who chose to become involved with Magdalene specifically because of the program's commitment to house the women without imposing residential staff or other live-in authority figures on them. She described the conflict:

> The tension in Magdalene has been and continues to be wanting to be a community about love and needing to be a place where people are safe. And in order for people to be safe, there do have to be some limits, and there has to be some authority. And, particularly the women that we bring in, certainly in their first year there, they need to know, they need some outer parameters. But I think what's different about Magdalene is that that isn't the whole program—it's a piece of what we provide.

Finally, the commitment to employ every Magdalene woman who needs a job for at least some length of time poses some obvious challenges to Thistle Farms as a fledgling company. First, the capacity of its workforce to make products often outweighs the demand for them, meaning that the director of Thistle Farms is constantly trying to find engaging work for the women to do beyond producing inventory. Among other things, "work" at Thistle Farms frequently includes computer classes, speaking engagements, and product development experiments. While these are worthwhile activities, they do not directly increase the income generated from making or selling products. Although Thistle Farms sells a fair amount of inventory for a small bath and body company, it does not currently sell enough to cover its operating expenses (most of which are consumed by labor costs), and therefore relies on grants and private donations to stay financially solvent.

Like other businesses operating this close to the margin of solvency, Thistle Farms makes hard choices in order to honor its primary commitment of providing employment. Indeed, the long-term plan for Thistle Farms is for it to grow large enough to employ all Magdalene residents and graduates who desire employment, and to compensate them with living wages and health benefits. At the present time, though, Thistle Farms can offer only part-time employment, and it does not provide health benefits. For the women who work at Thistle Farms while living at Magdalene, roughly $100 a week for fifteen hours of work is a viable income because their expenses are minimal; their purchases typically include cigarettes and other nonessential personal items.[2]

The Thistle Farms director and the members of its managing council work diligently to find ways to employ Magdalene graduates and to pay them enough to support their needs. Most graduates who work at Thistle Farms earn approximately ten dollars an hour, work twenty hours a week, and receive Medicaid and other government subsidies such as food stamps. This combination of wages and subsidies is typically "enough" for graduates who receive other support such as disability benefits, and for those who are married to or live with employed partners. For other graduates, however, finding employment apart from or in addition to their jobs at Thistle Farms is necessary.

Becca and Holli both named increased hours, wages, and benefits as top priorities in the coming years. Becca feels guilty that Thistle Farms employees are not paid more than they are; on the other hand, there are no resources for providing higher pay or benefits at this time.

Its beliefs and business practices are nontraditional in many senses, but like all businesses, Thistle Farms can remain open only as long as its income meets or exceeds its expenses. And as long as the company continues to be one of the few employers in Nashville providing jobs to women in recovery or with psychological disabilities, there will continue to be a large number of women seeking and needing work at Thistle Farms.

Offering Kindness

In April 2008, I traveled with Becca and four other women from the Magdalene community to a women's cooperative in Kigali, Rwanda. After what had been a remarkable visit, we stood in a slow-moving airport security line, exhausted and lost in thought over all that we had learned, seen, and experienced. As the line went from slow-moving to a standstill, people grew increasingly irritated at a young Rwandan woman at the front of the line who could not find her passport. She was traveling with a small child and multiple bags. Sensing the irritation behind her, she frantically tried to dig through her purse, all the while juggling her baby and her luggage. Everyone, including me, was wishing that the woman would pull herself together so we could get through security and begin our long journey home. As we stood watching, Becca left the line, approached the woman, and said, "Can I hold something for you?" The woman, relieved and grateful, handed her baby to Becca, set her bags down, and seconds later found her passport. I remember being at once touched and guilt-stricken over how simple it is to offer kindness to the people around us when we have eyes to see and the will to respond. In a sense, what Becca did for the woman in Rwanda is a snapshot of what the community of Magdalene House offers to the residents, graduates, staff, and volunteers who come through its doors: grace, kindness, reprieve, and moments of companionship for the many journeys that are too difficult to travel alone.

CHAPTER 6

Come as You Are

Love, Forgiveness, and Belonging

> The day that I found out that I really couldn't stop using
> without help, it scared me to death. And I started to
> believe the lie that I was going to die on those streets.
> Either a trick was going to take me out—because there
> had been many rapes, you know, I've been pushed out
> of cars and all kind of stuff. I've been kidnapped—and
> so I believed that if a trick didn't kill me, then I would
> probably hit a piece of dope and blow my heart up or
> something. But I believed that I was going to die that
> way.
>
> —Marion, Magdalene House graduate

WITH ANY ILLNESS COMES not only the actual physical or mental manifestation of disease, but also the way disease is interpreted. Years of study have demonstrated that the interpretation of pain and illness is as important as the disease itself in determining how sickness is experienced and treated. Sarah Coakley, a Cambridge philosopher and theologian who studies pain and embodiment, gives this example to illustrate how the interpretation of pain can affect the very experience of it: if you wake up with an unexplained, splitting headache on the tenth anniversary of your father's death from brain cancer, it *means* something different than if you wake up with a splitting headache after having a few too many glasses of wine the night before.

114

According to Coakley and many others, the dance between embodied symptoms on the one hand and meaning-making and interpretation on the other takes place for all experiences of illness and pain (Coakley and Shelemay 2007; Kleinman 1988). Furthermore, the interpretation of illness draws its power and meaning from the social and cultural contexts in which the sick individual exists. Perhaps nowhere is this truer than in the realm of mental illness.

The relationship between mental illness and shame has a long history, especially when it comes to addiction. Despite prevalence rates indicating that a substantial portion of the US population has or will experience mental illness at some time in their lives, and a culture increasingly open to conversations about addiction, there remains a belief that mental illness and substance abuse are private experiences that should be kept secret. Compounding this belief are attributions of addiction that ascribe "the problem" to individual factors such as personality traits and genetic makeup. Although locating the etiology of addiction in the physical body represents a more progressive view than previous notions that frame addiction as a moral deficit, it often still fails to acknowledge broader systems and relationships that inevitably contribute to the existence and experience of addiction. Furthermore, research demonstrates that biological (and particularly genetic) explanations for mental illness increasingly lead people to believe that illness will be persistent and untreatable throughout the course of their lives (Phelan, Yang, and Cruz-Rojas 2006).

Although it is unlikely that the women at Magdalene encountered neurobiological and genetic explanations of addiction while they were on the streets, the beliefs and narratives that accompany these explanations influence the social meaning of addiction. This meaning is ingested and reproduced through social and cultural institutions, with which the women at Magdalene, as well as the rest of us, come into constant contact. As such, the women at Magdalene did encounter beliefs and explanations of addiction, either from within themselves or from others, that affected their experience. Namely, the meaning-making processes that surround addiction told them: *You* are the problem, and the problem will *always* exist.

In addition to informing the beliefs we hold about addicted individuals, and that addicted individuals hold about themselves, dominant social narratives inform the way addiction is addressed and treated (Mulia 2002; Singer 2008). Furthermore, the service system most commonly accessed by persons of color who suffer from addiction is the justice system, which provides little opportunity for rehabilitation (Roberts 2000; Mulia 2002). In this sense, beliefs about drug use being persistent and criminal inform systems-level structures (such as drug laws and prison facilities) that recommend "punishment" as an adequate and appropriate treatment for addiction. In turn, individual experiences are shaped in such a way that the dominant narratives become real: women develop internal self-concepts that tell them they will never be more than addicts, prostitutes, felons, or throw-aways, and these self-concepts provide scripts for the way they live their lives.

Every woman I interviewed said, "I thought that I would always use," and most said, "I thought I would die because of it." Talking about living on the streets, Katie said, "I used to just think that I would be a crackhead for the rest of my life. That I would never do anything else." Similarly, Kristin said, "I've always known that I had a drug problem, but I always thought that I would just always use drugs, and that my life would always be fucked up. I just thought that it was going to be like that." Tricia, who had grown up in a better household than many, said that her early experiences with addiction made her feel "like I was a disappointment. I always thought that I was just a mess-up. That my parents didn't need no child like me. [But] I kept that to myself."

For most women at Magdalene, their experiences in prison, at other treatment centers, and with friends and families echoed the negative and degrading interpretations of addiction and illness. Furthermore, their illnesses and corresponding behaviors and experiences came accompanied by tremendous feelings of guilt and shame. Describing the weight of shame and its potential role in acting as a barrier to recovery, Tricia said:

> More than the scars that I carry on the outside, I'm still haunted by
> certain things that I seen on the streets. I'm telling you, and it's not
> even about the drugs. It wasn't—even though I was in my addiction,
> it wasn't about the drugs no more. I was caught up in the lifestyle, you

know what I'm saying? The going, the doing, the—whoever I wanted to hang with, you told me not to do something, I looked straight at you and said, "I'm fixin' to do it anyway." And I've seen a lot of stuff that you just ain't gonna live to tell somebody else about it. You know what I'm saying? These eyes have seen and witnessed a lot of stuff, and it haunts me today. And when I got to Magdalene, I thought, "How in the world am I going to deal with all the stuff that's going on inside me, live a recovery program, and still hold my head up?"

Similarly, Toni said:

When I first came into Magdalene, I didn't speak for three months, but I knew that it was something I had to do, so they just taught me to just say my name. I wouldn't even say my name for three months. I wouldn't even say hi to nobody. I guess because I was beating myself up for who I was and what I had done. Plus I had never really been in a program before. So, I didn't know what to expect. So I was kind of ashamed and kind of shy. It was kind of hard for me to just tell people where I had been, what I have done, and to hear myself say those things.

The beliefs about addiction reported by the women at Magdalene—that it is all-encompassing, untreatable, and worthy of shame and alienation—mean that an essential task in the healing work of Magdalene is to provide a safe community in which disease and illness can be reinterpreted. Using the language of brokenness, staff, women, and volunteers create an interpretation of illness that links disease to social, economic, and political structures as well as to individual and family characteristics. Furthermore, brokenness is a quality believed to be common to all people and communities, signaling a universal need for love and forgiveness rather than condemnation. Magdalene posits a view of illness in which suffering and awareness of human need serve as grounds for mystery, creativity, transformation, and hope—both for the self and for others. Through these formulations, Magdalene constructs and practices an interpretation of healing and health that implies connectedness and re-creation.

As stated before, these beliefs and commitments are more than window dressing. The very experience of illness and pain can be altered based on the individual and sociocultural interpretations of it (Kleinman 1988). Because the process of meaning-making and interpretation takes place in an ongoing negotiation between individuals and their sociocultural context or contexts, providing a community through which illness and disease are reinterpreted in fact changes the very nature and experience of illness itself.

Meanings of Brokenness

Not long after I began volunteering at Thistle Farms, I was making copies of product order forms when Gina walked up to use the copy machine for her shipping orders. While we waited for my batch to finish, we chatted. Gina asked me how old I was and what I was learning in school and if I had a boyfriend. When I told her I was twenty-nine, she gasped and said, "See, I love that, because my daughter is twenty-nine. And that means we're like, the *same.*" Through most people's eyes, there were few similarities between Gina and me beyond the fact that we were both, at that moment, standing at the copy machine. Gina is an elderly African American woman who grew up on the streets of Knoxville, Tennessee. Her mother was a sex worker and a drug addict, just like Gina, and just like Gina's daughter. Gina has never had much formal education. She is bald, missing fingers on each of her hands, and reliant on an oxygen tank most of the time. She has experienced violence and racism and poverty that I, as a white, well-educated, middle-class woman whose life has mostly been marked by safety and privilege, will probably never experience. Gina is also an incredible artist (an ability to which I have long aspired, but feel certain I will never attain), a powerful speaker, and a listener. She hears the voice of God with a certainty and clarity that makes me doubt the strength of my own faith (or, perhaps, the strength of my own doubts). I think that I would have felt naive and ignorant afterward had I ever said to Gina, "See . . . we're the same."

But when Gina went on to explain her claim of sameness, she told me something that shaped the rest of my experience at Magdalene, as well as my relationships in the community and my approach to understanding healing and recovery. Gina said, "Before I came to Magdalene, I always believed that people like me weren't as valuable as people like you. I was raised to believe that people like me shouldn't talk to people like you. That people like me don't belong in the same room as people like you. But you know what I've learned? I've learned that that's a *lie*. Because I've learned that we're all broken, and I've learned that we're all valuable."

The claims that "we're all broken" and "we're all valuable" are metaphysical claims as much as any other. They rely on an idea (supported with ample evidence) of human fragility and need, partnered with a belief that human life — each human life — is sacred and worthy of dignity and respect. It also means that each person needs others and is needed *by* others in the journey toward healing, whether the person is an "addict" or a "counselor" or a "volunteer." This idea is foreign to the traditional culture of healing that envisions professionals as expert healers and patients as bodies on which professionals work their expert magic. It is also foreign, one might argue, to the somewhat more progressive culture that envisions professionals and clients as "partners," particularly because acknowledging brokenness as an ongoing quality of *all* involved parties tends to lend itself poorly to a well-ordered, well-defined, forward-moving partnership.

While Magdalene does rely heavily and gratefully on the services of professional healers such as doctors, dentists, nurses, and psychologists to treat and care for the women who join the community, it also operates out of a belief that the community itself makes full healing possible. Speaking to the importance of community as both the cause and the solution to the illnesses experienced by women at Magdalene, Becca said, "It's a story of brokenness and a community breaking down. All the stories we hear of the women, we've got families breaking down, school systems breaking down, church systems breaking down, penal systems breaking down. And so it takes a broken community to make sure the women get on the streets, it's going to take that same community to get women off the streets."

Although understanding the world and self as broken might seem alienating to some, for the residents, staff, and volunteers who find their place in the Magdalene circle, the belief is tremendously liberating. It means that imperfection is inevitable and common. It means that the brokenness in my story might speak to the brokenness in your story, and for that reason I should share my story instead of hide it. It means that we all need forgiveness and have grounds to seek it for ourselves and offer it to others. It means that regardless of cultural narratives of autonomy and individuality, we are not sufficient unto ourselves. Paradoxically, the narrative of brokenness also means we all belong to a common human family: a family in which each member is worthy of being loved and loving others.

Love and Belonging: Reinterpreting the Addicted Self

The relationship between brokenness and belonging is perhaps best illustrated by the hospitality the community of Magdalene offers to outsiders and newcomers, be they women coming off the streets or new volunteers. Jenny, a volunteer at Thistle Farms, talked about coming to Magdalene after having spent a long time in a corporate environment:

> I think the key thing is to be valued for who you are. I think that's very healing, and that's what I get here. I feel like I'm valued for who I am, warts and all. And allowing people to be themselves, I think that frees them from the bondage of their past. You don't have to . . . people don't care about the bad things that I did. And that's very freeing to me, to know that they'll accept me even if I sit here and say, "I did this, I did that" or whatever, and they'll love me anyways.

This openness and hospitality is equally important for the women who come to Magdalene from the streets. Because addiction and illness has so often meant alienation and isolation for the women at Magdalene, providing a community in which they feel loved and accepted is an essential step in the path to recovery. Women report that the often painful and vulnerable process of healing is possible only within the context of unconditional relationships that suspend judgment and offer forgiveness. Kayla said:

> When I first got to Magdalene, everything was pretty cloudy. Having been on the streets, and not eating, not sleeping, not even bathing, my mind was pretty cloudy, and I was afraid because I didn't think that the program would work, but I was desperate, so I was willing to try anything. And when I got there, I remember walking into a community meeting and the women greeted me like they had known me all my life. And these women were total strangers to me, and they began to put their arms around me and hug me and were telling me, "Come on in, girl," and I was like, "Wow," 'cause it was totally different from where I had come from — the streets — where you sleep with one eye open and one eye closed. But they welcomed me in and they began to pamper me, and the first couple of weeks that I was there, I just rested.

Along with the safety and hospitality offered by the community, most women say they came to Magdalene, stayed at Magdalene, and healed at Magdalene because of the love offered to them there. While sitting on the old, dingy couches at Thistle Farms one day, I asked Kathleen, "What is it about Magdalene that helped you heal?" She thought for a moment and replied: "Unconditional love. They didn't want anything. I didn't have to pay anything. The price was, how much was I willing to give myself? . . . It's not fake. It's real. People who love me no matter where I've come from. No matter what I've done." To emphasize the point, she said:

> I can remember, I think I was like a week clean, or eight days clean. And everybody — this was before I met Becca — everybody was hugging her and they were laughing, and I was like, "Who is this lady? Why is everybody hugging her?" And I remember she got close to me, and I was like, "I'm not gonna let her hug me because I'm still smellin'." And she reached over and she hugged me and she wouldn't let me go. And that was what I had been looking for all my life. I just cried.

All the women I interviewed told stories like Kathleen's—stories about being brought into a community of women who affirmed their value and common humanity by welcoming them with open arms. Katie said:

> There was just so much love in the program that they make you feel right at home, you know. They don't judge you, and that's the staff and the women. So I felt really comfortable when I came in. And I loved it. When I first came into Magdalene, I was such—I wanted people to like me so much that I was a people pleaser. I would do anything to make them happy, and I wasn't building any relationships. And so when I finally started to relax and be myself, I began to build relationships. And I do have a lot of relationships with the women in the program. And even the new women that come in, I try to, like, show them the same love I was shown when I came in, so they'll feel at home and comfortable and not want to leave.

It would be easy to interpret the Magdalene community as an unrealistic, Pollyanna version of illness and recovery. Practices such as "love" and "hospitality" are difficult to accomplish when they are truly extended to all, and many have argued that positive emotions and feel-good service do little to bring about the lasting, political changes that would name illness as a problem of injustice (McKnight 1995; Prilleltensky and Nelson 2002). While these are certainly concerns of which to be aware, Joel Shuman and Keith Meador (2003) propose framing the politics of care somewhat differently. In their book *Heal Thyself*, they argue that "in the world of the acquisitive, self-interested individual, illness is a threat because it hinders the pursuit of individual goods. Sick people cannot work or enjoy the fruits of their work, and their sickness is typically understood as a burden on those (nonprofessionals) who care for them" (130). In this sense, providing love and hospitality to those who are sick is in and of itself an opportunity for political transformation, because it specifically poses a different view of the ends and purposes of human life. "Illness and caring for illness are thus always fundamentally political acts" because "the primary threat posed by illness is not that it threatens to destroy the body of the person, although that is certainly a legitimate concern that must be addressed, but that it alienates the ill member from those other members of the community on whom she is dependent for life's greatest (nonmaterial) goods" (130). Furthermore, Shuman and Meador observe that the profound challenges of being sick and caring for the sick require the formation of communities through which the values of mercy and forgiveness can be developed and practiced.

Forgiveness as Transformation

Among other things, the practice of forgiveness provides a mechanism through which women can lay down old burdens and begin to work on new concepts of self. When women learn to forgive themselves, they find that the process of self-forgiveness is deeply connected to offering forgiveness to others and perceiving forgiveness from God. Indeed, forgiveness of self, forgiveness of others, and perceived forgiveness from God are interwoven and necessary ingredients in the journey toward healing. It is somewhat telling that the stories of forgiveness and healing that the women offer mirror those of soldiers and others in post-conflict areas more than they do the traditional literature on health and forgiveness. For the women at Magdalene, forgiveness is challenging work that involves revisiting egregious wrongs—wrongs they enacted, and wrongs done to them.

When I began exploring the concept of forgiveness and its relationship to healing, I thought about it in much the same way that it is presented in the academic literature—that forgiveness is good for one's mental and physical health, that forgiveness can be either a one-time act or an ongoing personal disposition, and that forgiveness has different dimensions depending on who is offering it and to whom it is being offered. While these divisions and categories have proven to be useful in scientific studies of the effects of forgiveness on health, forgiveness as the women at Magdalene described it is a much more mysterious and tangled experience that defies neat categories. For example, when

I asked Marion to talk a little bit about forgiveness and healing, she said:

> I think a lot of women felt like I felt—that I'd never be able to be a mother again, that my children are not going to forgive me. I'm not going to be able to listen to them or hear the pain that I've caused them. Because it's like we lost our humanness out there. We became just survivors of the street—of the wild. Either you trick, or you're gonna be tricked. Either you use, or you're gonna be used. My plan was always to get them before they got me. And it's like, because of all the abuse, I became an abuser—to anybody, it didn't matter. And coming into Magdalene, it just turned everything, you know? I'm still amazed at how God loved me, in spite of my rebellion. Even today. He has loved me through it all. He's not let go of me, and he's put people in my life, being interested for whatever reason. Just to talk about it helps the healing—you know, the slow process of healing comes about much faster. Forgiveness is part of the healing, and there's a process of healing, that will probably go on forever, because of everything that happened . . . but I'm able to because of Magdalene. And it's all related, you know: we get set up with therapists, something that we probably would have never done on the streets, or with medical help that we probably would have never done on the streets—too busy getting high, can't quit the corner, you know. We were able to go back to school, we were able to go back and get job skills . . . [and] learn how to be a person again. I got my kids back. That's the most important thing.

Marion's testimony about healing and forgiveness tells us that forgiveness is an ongoing process, involves multiple parties, relies on the support of others, and often requires real, tangible services to buttress the work of reconciling relationships with self, others, and God. Offering a similar account of the messy but powerful role of forgiveness in healing, Kathleen said:

> Once I found out that I wasn't alone, that I didn't have to walk through the pain by myself, it got easier. I started dealing with the

molestation, I started dealing with the abandonment, I started facing my fears. When I had sixty days clean, I was able to go back to Columbia [Tennessee], and confront the guy that molested me. I was face to face with him, and when I asked him why he took my childhood from me, the only thing he could say was, "I'll pay you this time." I couldn't run. And I wanted to. I wanted to go to get high. I wanted to numb the feelings that I was feeling, but I knew that I had to forgive him. I knew that he didn't know what he had done to me. And the day that I forgave him, my process started. Because I had to look back at all the things that I had done to my kids, to the people that loved me, and if God can forgive me, why I can't forgive him? And by me forgiving him, I was able to forgive myself. And I was able to move on, you know? Be healthy. Be free. It hasn't been an easy journey, but this journey is better than the journey that I lived. I wouldn't give this journey up for nothing in the world. I'm grateful. I'm very, very, very grateful to be able to talk about the pain. What's freedom for me? It's going back, reliving those deep dark secrets that I said that I was going to take to my grave. Freedom is letting somebody else know that they are not the only one that has done something, or has been in places that you told yourself that you never wanted to go, and find yourself there anyway. Freedom is allowing somebody to see the struggle that you went through, and allowing them not to live in the pit of hell. Freedom is knowing that, when you have been wrong, that God loves me anyway.

At the advice of several in the Magdalene community, I interviewed Father Charlie Strobel, founder of the Campus for Human Development in Nashville, while conducting my research for this book. Father Strobel has spent more than twenty years working with men and women living on the streets of Nashville, as well as fighting for the political changes that he believes are necessary to truly address the existence of homelessness. When I went to meet with Father Strobel, I was unable to find a place to park at the campus, so I parked across the street in front of a local business. To be polite—and also to forestall having my car towed—I went into the business to ask permission to leave my car while in my meeting. The woman at the desk generously allowed me to take up a spot in her parking lot, but she also expressed genuine concern about where I was going. "You *know* there are homeless people over there?" she asked, partly scolding. I assured her that I knew, and that someone would be there to meet me. I felt simultaneously comforted and repelled by her concern.

Over the course of the next few minutes, I learned my own important lesson about forgiveness. As I crossed the street and walked under an exhaust-stained overpass, I felt the men on the corner take notice of me, and then began to hear their taunts: "Hey girl, where you goin'?" "You got somethin' for me today?" "You probably shouldn't be down here by yourself—you know we'll get ya, ha ha ha ha." At that moment, I felt more angry than threatened but could not tease out who, exactly, I was angry with. I was angry with the men for making me feel scared and stupid. I was angry with myself for being angry with them, and for being angry with the woman in the store whom I had judged "judgmental," now knowing that she had probably endured this very experience hundreds of times. I also felt a bigger anger: an anger at injustice. An anger that stemmed from the realization that at the end of the day, I would most likely make it to my meeting, conduct my interview, get back in my car, drive back to my house, eat a healthy and filling dinner, and sleep in a warm bed. The men, on the other hand, would be on the streets during my meeting, during my drive home, during my dinner, and during my good night's sleep. In the story of life in Nashville, these men are a corner of the backdrop, like the women at Magdalene once were—neither invited to participate in the story nor to have their voices heard.

What I learned about forgiveness that day is that, at least in situations like these, the brokenness and interconnectedness of even seemingly disparate existences make it difficult to forgive any unless we "forgive it all" (Women of Magdalene 2008, 51). This does not mean that "anything goes," of course: I would rather not feel threatened while walking down the street, and I would rather live in a world in which homelessness is unthinkable, because to have people living in such inhumane circumstances represents a failure of decency on all our parts. What it does mean is that making sense of the anger to figure out whom to blame is tremendously tiring, and probably doesn't move me (or them) much further on the road to justice and healing.

Once I got closer to the campus and the men on the corner, I decided to answer them. I called out, "I'm here to see Father Strobel."

The apparent leader of the men responded, "Well, why didn't you say so earlier? I'm Stephen, and Charlie Strobel is a good man." Stephen escorted me into the campus and took me to Father Strobel's office. As promised by the women at Magdalene, the interview was well worth my time. Father Strobel offered an insightful historical perspective on Magdalene as an organization, and affirmed many of my observations about the qualities and practices of Magdalene that make it a healing community. Linking brokenness, acceptance, and forgiveness on the path to healing, he said:

> Healing is more than just physical healing. And of course there's a lot of that that has to occur because [the women's] bodies are broken, bruised, abused, and their bodies have been weakened over the years from drug use, living outdoors, and so everybody needs a time to heal, physically. There's a lot of mental and emotional healing that has to occur. And people aren't able to do that as easily with a twenty-day treatment center or a thirty-day treatment center, because all it does is dry you out. Thirty days and you never really come to terms with the stuff that's inside of you—all the stuff—toxic stuff. . . . People here, people in Magdalene, they need a place where they can dump all that toxicity. So in a sense, this place and Magdalene both allow people to dump all that toxicity, and that takes a long time. And to be able to do that without suffering recriminations, without being judged, is a tremendous grace. And it's the grace of healing, and the grace of healing is the grace of forgiveness.

When she described her process of healing at Magdalene, Kayla echoed Father Strobel's explanation of the need for a community where time, companionship, and forgiveness are in ample supply:

> I began to see the girls doing some of our program groups, and I was watching them and I was listening to them talk about stuff that had

happened, and I was like, "Wow. I'm not the only one. I'm not the only one that this has happened to. I'm not the only one that has done some of this horrible stuff." And, I began to just kind of ease in and sit in on groups also, and before I knew it, you know, I was in. Right in doing what everybody else was doing: talking, sharing, learning how to heal.

Contrasting this with other treatment programs she had been through, she said:

I think the longest time I stayed in a regular treatment center was maybe six months, and the twenty-eight day, the forty-five day, the ninety days, for me, it was just not enough time to get my head clear and decide that I did want to stay clean, and to actually . . . do some intense therapy, to actually get to the root of why I was using. I didn't wake up one day and decide, "I want to be a junkie. I want to be a prostitute." There were things that led me to that. And I had to kind of relive some of those things in therapy in order to deal with them. And I had to relive 'em, and I had to talk about 'em. Had to cry about 'em. And Magdalene provides us with therapists: trained professionals that are able to open those wounds, and then close 'em back up. Magdalene is a safe place.

The perception that Magdalene is a safe place cannot be underestimated when talking about key ingredients for healthy recovery. The psychiatrist and medical anthropologist Arthur Kleinman (1998) writes about the importance of "witnessing and helping to order" (xii) patient stories as they experience illness and seek healing. According to this formulation, allowing people to talk about their experiences with illness—even experiences that cannot be changed—serves the purpose of authenticating and making meaning in the lives of those who suffer. Although there are not easy explanatory models through which to interpret or put in order the pain of abuse or the shame of addiction, bearing witness and finding out that others share similar pain has profound transformative power.

Healing and Re-creation: Developing New Notions of Self

At Magdalene, talking about illness and bearing witness is a practice that is central to the community. Most often, the practice takes place through storytelling, or more specifically, "telling one's story." There are many forms of storytelling and multiple narrative frames represented in the tradition of storytelling at Magdalene, not the least of which is the twelve-step tradition of recovery. Within the twelve-step tradition, individuals come together to hold one another accountable and take steps toward recovery, often by sharing past experiences and current struggles with one another (SAMHSA 2006). Women living in the Magdalene houses are encouraged to have group meditation once a day at a time of their choosing, during which they set aside twenty to thirty minutes to read a passage from a twelve-step text and share their thoughts about the passage or anything else that might be of immediate importance for their recovery. At Thistle Farms, a similar meditation is held at the beginning of each workday, and includes anyone visiting, volunteering, or working at the company. This meditation is often referred to as "the circle," which is an apt description: everyone participating in it shows up at 9:00 a.m. and pulls up a folding chair, forming a large circle that fills the main room at Thistle Farms. Its members vary from day to day, but the practice stays the same: a Magdalene resident or graduate reads the meditation for the day, which is chosen from a variety of sources. Then the participants work their way around the circle, one by one, each person reflecting on what had been read or, often, the community in general. Twelve-step mantras such as "just for today," "you spot it, you got it," "the God of my understanding," and "a grateful addict is a recovering addict" are commonplace. In addition to being practices that the women say help their recovery, the circle and other twelve-step rituals provide places for confession, truth-telling, and identity reconstruction that the women find healing. Recalling one particularly memorable meeting, Kayla told me:

I can tell you what my first sense of freedom was for me. It was when I began to talk about being HIV positive. That was like this huge load was lifted from my shoulders, because for probably about five or six years, I lived in this world trying to keep everybody that knew me from knowing that I was HIV positive. And I had conjured up all this stuff in my head about what people would think, and what people would say, and how people would treat me. And I remember the first time I talked about it, I was in a meeting, I thought my heart was going to stop beating. But people's reactions were not what I thought they would be, and it was just a relief.

For Kayla, the ability to tell her story provided freedom because she was able to confront her fears and expectations of isolation and rejection. Like Kayla, many women at Magdalene are afflicted with mental and physical conditions other than addiction that are particularly alienating. Diseases such as depression, bipolar disorder, schizophrenia, HIV-related infections, and hepatitis C have long-term embodied symptoms that often lead to great suffering. Similar to addiction, these diseases also have implications for interpersonal relationships and carry social meanings that influence how and when a person is accepted and integrated into the communities that surround them. That people in the community were supportive of Kayla, rather than fearful or condemning, allowed her disclosure to be healing. Furthermore, she told me that the healing that came from this experience was the one that encouraged her to talk more openly with her therapist and to deal with some of the issues underlying her drug use. For many of the women, the presence of an open and accepting community provided a place where they could dispose of secrets and old narratives that had haunted them for years. Talking about her experience with telling her story, Michelle said:

I started telling my story and the first time that I was able to tell the big secret that I had never told anybody and got that much freedom from it, then I became willing to do it again because I've been toting this stuff and I've been miserable and nobody judged me and everybody is still OK with me. And the more I told it, the less power it had, you know, so it started becoming a selfish thing to me. You know what I'm saying? I want to do this, you know, I want to get better, because I've been toting this stuff for thirty or forty years.

In addition to providing a safe and supportive environment where women can lay down the secrets and burdens they have carried for decades, the circle provides the opportunity to create, claim, and be held accountable to new notions of the self. Julian Rappaport uses the framework of community narratives to help make sense of stories and practices that shape individual and collective identity. Narratives, as discussed by Rappaport (1995, 2000), are the stories we use to define ourselves. They tell us "not only who we are but who we have been and who we can be" (1995, 796). These narratives affect individuals by creating meaning and influencing emotion, memory, and identity; however, they exist on many levels of analysis (individual, organizational, community) and all these levels influence each other (1995). Narratives are created, re-created, and internalized or manifested through a constant interplay of dominant cultural narratives, community narratives, and individual narratives (1995, 2000) These narratives can be true or untrue, positive or negative, or constructive or harmful, and work together to form the identities and inform the behaviors of the people and communities who create, transmit, and interact with them.

Although the women at Magdalene drew on numerous sources for their re-creations, beliefs in God were deeply integral to their new identities. When the women I interviewed told me their life stories and described their processes of recovery, they talked about the importance of prayer and meditation and coming to their own understanding of God in addition to working through issues of abuse, addiction, and trauma through more clinical means. Women talked about the importance of finding a God who was not their "grandmama's God." Women told me that they had found God in the back of cop cars, in deserted alleys, in prison cells, and in friendships with other addicts. To them, this meant that God was present in darkness as well as light, and it enabled them to construct an identity of someone cared for, accompanied and empowered regardless of circumstance, rather than cast off and alone. Explaining this process, Kathleen said, "Coming into Magdalene, I never had any discipline before. They taught me how to find myself. They taught me how to look deep within. They taught me how to find my own God—not my mom's god, not my grandmama's god, not that God that they said was going to come from the sky and beat me down. But I finally found a God that was loving, caring, forgiving, and compassionate."

As described by Kathleen and others, the process of finding one's own God was facilitated not only by the twelve-step tradition, but also by the spiritual leadership provided by Becca. Personal, spiritual discovery is encouraged at Magdalene, and Becca's unconventional style seems to enable residents, graduates, and volunteers to embrace the process in a way that is healing and freeing. After describing her resistance to Magdalene because it was a "religious" program headed by "some damn priest," Marion told me about the first time she met Becca:

> She had on some Daisy Duke shorts and a midriff top and her hair was just—I mean, she was like one of us, you know what I'm saying? And I was just like, "Oh my God—she's not a priest!" You know what I'm saying—priests do not dress like that. And it was just like overwhelming and it was just like love just oozed from her. It was just like, it is OK for you to be who you are. It is OK and we're going to walk with you for everything that you—whatever you want to do. As long as it's positive. And you don't have to go back and sell your body, you don't have to go back and use any dope, you don't have to let anybody abuse or use you. We're gonna help you walk into your life. And I was just like, in . . . shock, just looking at this woman, and I was just amazed that she doesn't look like a priest. But then what does a priest look like? And I say all the time that Becca reminds me of the Lord. She reminds me of Jesus. You know, it's just like standin' there: just come as you are. We're going to walk with you and we love you and I mean it was *genuine*. And it still is.

Although I have never seen Becca dressed quite as Marion described, she is certainly unlike any priest I have ever encountered.

More importantly, her ability to inspire people to find their own path and walk on it is remarkable. Members of the Magdalene community find it to be a place of inclusion, forgiveness, and creativity. Holli, the director of Thistle Farms, spoke of the absence of "cookie cutter" expectations:

> We all can find ourselves on different paths of our spiritual journey, and to find yourself on whatever journey that is. I remember Toni saying, "I don't know that I believe in God." And it was very freeing to be in a place that wasn't like, "What do you mean, you don't believe in God?!" The response was like, "Yeah, I've been there before, too." It was just very, like—wow—I could breathe or something.

Clearly, the imagery of being on a journey is central to the processes of self- and spiritual discovery at Magdalene. Among other things, this metaphor allows individual members and the community as a whole the freedom to look at themselves and say, "I'm not there yet . . . we're not there yet . . . but we're on our way." The identity constructed by such a narrative is healing because it allows for and embraces imperfection and re-creation. As I heard many times at Magdalene, it means that "the only thing that matters is showing up and being a part of" the community. Ali, a divinity student who works for Magdalene, talked about this aspect of the community in her interview:

> Something that stands out to me is . . . the drive of the people who participate, the people who volunteer, the people who are staff members, the women who are in the program. We are reading Niebuhr in one of my classes and we were talking about how, basically, you're going to have dirty hands. Like, you're not going to go into something able to do what is right, like completely what is right—you're going to have dirty hands. And I think that that is acknowledged—you can kind of come as you are. . . . There is still a yearning to do something. Like you're going to have dirty hands, but that doesn't mean that you shouldn't do something.

Along with the journey metaphor, the stories that were told again and again are messages of hope and healing. During one particularly memorable meditation at Thistle Farms, I witnessed the power that language has to shape the mood and identity of a community. In the week preceding the meditation, several painful things had happened at Magdalene: a graduate who worked at Thistle Farms had relapsed and no one could find her or contact her, two other women had learned that their mothers had cancer, and it seemed as though the newly re-designed Thistle Farms products were not going to be ready in time to meet the deadline for their launch with an advertising company in New York. The weight of the losses, fears, and disappointments was tangible as the women went around the circle and responded to the day's meditation. One of the women said, "I feel like everywhere I look, there is death and darkness all around me."

When it was Becca's turn to speak, she acknowledged the legitimacy of everyone's feelings, but then said that she was not discouraged—that her time with the Magdalene community had taught her never to give up hope on people or on situations, even when things seem desperate. She went on to say that addiction would not have the last word on Suzanne, that death will not have the last word on any of us, and that the circle itself was a testament to the truth that in the end, love wins. Her words changed the atmosphere of the entire community—moods were better, relationships were stronger, and productivity was higher.

Among other things, this situation illustrates the power of narrative to construct and to reinterpret. Whether or not Becca's words were "true" or "untrue" when she spoke them is of little importance—they became true once they were spoken, which is the lesson that theories of narrative and social construction offer. Furthermore, Nancy Hirschmann (2003) warns against an understanding of social construction in which we envision an *un*constructed self or society. Rather, she says, everything is always already constructed and interpreted. Because Hirschmann is a political theorist concerned with freedom, she would say that our challenge is to look for holes in oppressive discourses in order to reshape them into discourses of liberation. For the women in the community of Magdalene, one of the challenges of healing is reconstructing the discourses and understandings of illness that keep people sick. Seemingly greatest among these is the idea of illness as an individual experience that manifests itself only in the body or mind. Beliefs such as these tell us that illness and healing are both the responsibility of individuals and professional service providers, and that community is something to be joined after one is well. In contrast, by interpreting illness as brokenness and a need for membership, the community of Magdalene House offers a narrative of healing that requires relationships marked by love, forgiveness, and belonging.

CHAPTER 7

Speaking Our Truth in Love

Each time I tell my story, it's healing for me. And what I have noticed is that every time I go somewhere and I share my story, somebody comes to me afterwards and says, "I have a daughter . . ." or "I have a sister . . ." or "I struggle with . . ." or "I'm in recovery . . ." So I know that me speaking my truth helps other people tap into their own truth, and that's what it's all about—me sharing what I've been through to help somebody else get through what they're going through. And I guess I just hope that my healing process is attractive to other women and other people, and that sharing it makes them want to heal also.

—Kayla, Magdalene House graduate

JUST AS SHARING STORIES is a healing practice within the Magdalene House community, sharing stories with other communities, organizations, and funders serves an important purpose as well. Spreading "the message of Magdalene" entails speaking at public events, publishing written material, and positing a vision of health and flourishing in which "no one is left to be condemned," and it is "always wrong to buy and sell women." Magdalene's messages are anti-prostitution and pro-recovery, and they appeal to a communal sense of responsibility for the suffering and healing of others. In addition to combating discourses about addiction and prostitution that they perceive to be destructive, members of the community believe that speaking about Magdalene has the power to cast a vision for what the world *could* be: a place where people love without judgment, care for their neighbors, support one another regardless of circumstance, and defend human dignity.

Practices of Speaking

In 2008, Magdalene residents and graduates spoke at over 180 events. Although most of the engagements took place in the Nashville area, the women also spoke to audiences in Kansas City, Atlanta, New York, Chicago, and Orlando. The events varied in nature and audience, but were usually hosted by groups connected to some aspect of Magdalene's mission. Faith communities, university classrooms, local businesses, and women's groups heard the story of Magdalene, as did individuals attending Thistle Farms home parties in Nashville.

Typically, the stories that the women at Magdalene share follow a standard pattern: the speaker briefly recounts her experiences of being addicted, prostituting, and on the streets, then talks about entering the community of Magdalene, and ends with what her life looks like now. Michael Young (2007) describes how stories such as these capitalize on narratives of confession and conversion that are familiar to hearers in a culture that has been shaped by Judeo-Christian ideology. The Magdalene community is one of many organizations that use confession and conversion narratives to motivate change. These types of narratives gained political utility as early as the 1830s, when activists employed them to advocate for a variety of reforms, ranging from temperance to abolition. In particular, stories told by former slaves turned abolitionists closely mirror the stories of the women at Magdalene, in terms of reformers telling stories of victimization that are also about strength and survival. Furthermore, like former slaves, survivors of addiction, prostitution, and life on the streets ironically occupy a somewhat privileged position, at least in social locations where such persons are visible and included as part of the community, because of their personal knowledge of such aberrant experiences. Ownership of this type of information gives storytellers a certain type of power and authority, and when told in the context of a conversion narrative, said authority is also moral. Describing this phenomenon in slave narratives, Francesca Polletta (2006) argues, "The assumption was that the story itself would educate the moral intuitions of the reader (or hearers) in a way that would compel right action. On the template of the Christian conversation narrative, then, slave narrators were moral guides. They were victims, but also heroes" (115).

This phenomenon was evident during a meeting between Becca Stevens, a seasoned graduate of the Magdalene program, and the mayor of Nashville. Becca and the graduate, Kayla, were talking with Mayor Dean about the city providing Thistle Farms with an abandoned building so that the company could relocate to a larger, much needed space. While sitting in the mayor's office, high up in a government building in downtown Nashville, Mindy looked out the window and saw a run-down motel to which she used to go with "dates." Mindy called the experience "surreal" and felt it was representative of how far she has come since her time on the streets. Tellingly, she seemed undaunted by the semi-celebrity status that has been accorded to her as a result of her connections with Magdalene, nor did she appear particularly impressed that within a single moment, she could see and claim authority of experience in two places that most Nashvillians will never encounter—turning a trick in a seedy motel and sitting in Karl Dean's office. Mindy's experiences have allowed her to speak to issues of healing and justice in a way that goes beyond conventional understandings, and she sees advocacy for these issues as part of the responsibility of her experience with healing.

In the fall of 2009, with funding from a private foundation, Magdalene expanded its speaking schedule from churches and schools to women's prisons throughout the United States. The "prison tour" consisted of visits to eight women's prisons in eight different cities over the course of ten months. At each stop on the tour, residents and graduates from Magdalene shared stories about their lives before, during, and after the streets; two Nashville-based musicians performed; and Becca talked about Magdalene's theology of brokenness and healing. Going into a prison was not new to most of the residents and graduates, but Kayla described how she found herself in unfamiliar territory nonetheless:

I mean, I've been in prison before, but never while I was clean. Since I've been clean, I'm used to going into churches or other groups and talking to people who understand about healing—or who are at least friendly to the idea, you know? But you go into a prison, where most of the women in there are just—that's the last thing that's on their mind. Or at least that was the last thing on *my* mind when I was there. But when we talk about healing, there seems to be a glimmer of hope. There's a glimmer that maybe their thought process has been changed just a little bit—that maybe they're starting to believe that life can be different for them, too.

Speaking in the prisons was rewarding, says Kayla, but it was also hard work. She described a particularly difficult experience when the group spoke at Rikers Island prison in New York City:

When we left Rikers, it was so *heavy*. We got out of there, we were just drained. When we got to the airport, everybody was looking around at each other like, "Did we just . . . ?" "Yeah, we did." That was one of the hardest situations that we had to be in, because the women were totally close-minded. They didn't think that they wanted us there at first. They were booing us and yelling at us, but we just kept telling our stories, and the musicians kept playing, and we just kept pushing though. At the end, they were clapping and wanting to talk to us, and hugging on us, so it was like, it was worth it. It was just so draining.

What makes speaking in public on behalf of Magdalene "worth it" is not an uninteresting or unimportant question. According to the ethicist Stacey Floyd-Thomas (2006), when people tell their stories, they are telling stories of the present and future as well as the past. They present their past through an interpretive narrative structure that allows them to make sense of their lives in terms of where they've been, where they are, and where they're going. Inherent in this type of narrative is a notion of telos—an end, a goal—and an ethical assessment of how past experiences are contributing to notions of purpose and rightness. The past is remembered through the lens of the present, and the present is interpreted as a production of the past. This is not to say that the stories and recollections are inaccurate, but rather that they are neither objective nor concrete. Furthermore, the standards of objectivity and concreteness are not the appropriate standards to apply. Instead, the dynamic stories that people tell should be understood as representations of what has happened in the past, and how those happenings influence and are influenced by the creation of the self and experiences of the self's world in the present.

By telling stories about their own lives and the relationships, places, and experiences in and through which they have lived, women at Magdalene create, perform, and share their beliefs about themselves, the world, and the kind of lives worth living. Through the performance and sharing of stories of recovery, they are able to reinterpret the things that have happened to them and the things they've done in such a way that their experiences have purpose and significance. When audiences are receptive, these feelings of purpose and significance are reaffirmed. For example, Kathleen told me that sharing her story with outside audiences reminds her of who she is and how far she's come: "I love telling my story because that's where I came from, but that's not who I am. That's not the person that I am. That was bad choices that I made in life, you know?" She also believes telling her story helps other people heal and have hope, particularly those dealing with addiction and prostitution: "We just don't know how powerful our stories could be to a person that don't have a clue about what addiction and prostitution is, and they always got this lie that nobody never recovers, or they gonna be that way all their life, and we, we givin' them that hope shot, so our stories is important. No matter what kind of story you have, it's important, because you never know who needs to hear it."

Many of the women say that the ability to believe that they have something positive and healing to contribute to the world is an essential part of their recovery, and one of the many building blocks for constructing a valuable and useful self. Furthermore, believing that the suffering they have endured has meaning helps them, like many others, recontextualize and reinterpret their pain from something senseless to something generative (Das 2001). The women speak of wanting to use their stories to encourage other addicts and family members of addicts, to challenge dominant discourses about prostitution and the use of women's bodies, and to destigmatize mental illness. There is at least anecdotal evidence that these speaking strategies have had their intended effects. In the two years I worked at Thistle Farms, countless people (usually women) shuffled through the door just in time for meditation, timidly inquiring, "Is this Thistle Farms?" and "May I join you today?" They would then sit in the meditation circle and share that they were there because they had heard someone speak at an event, which had reminded them to keep fighting for a husband, daughter, sister, or son wrestling with addiction (often one who had "failed so many times"). Or they shared that they too were struggling with addiction, an abusive partner, mental illness, or feelings of shame and guilt. Outsiders said they came to Magdalene because they believed that people would listen to their stories with love and without judgment. They stayed because they found a community in which stories of brokenness were also stories of belonging and potential.

Breaking the Myths

Kayla, who is now the sales manager at Thistle Farms, believes that in addition to healing the self and helping others, telling her story can challenge broader cultural narratives, which she calls "myths," saying:

> I get to travel all over the world to talk about and break the myths about prostitution, addiction, and how there are enough places for women to recover, because there are not—there are not enough places for women to come, and feel safe, and deal with some of the issues that have led us to the streets. And to break the myths that once a prostitute, always a prostitute; once an addict, always an addict: No—we heal. We heal, we grow, and we move on.

The myths that the women from Magdalene are combating are not imagined. They have heard them from relatives, police officers, staff from other recovery programs, and through the media. Sherri told me about the woman who dropped her off at Magdalene when she decided to leave the streets: the woman, a representative from the courts, took Sherri to Magdalene, walked her in the front door, and yelled down the hall to Sonya, "Good luck with this one. She thinks she can live clean, but I know she can't. She'll be on and off the streets for life." Sherri said she used that insult to motivate her recovery on the days she wanted to turn back. Six years later, Sherri is still clean, and she has never once gone back to the streets.

Sherri's experience may have had something to do with the fact that she *had* been in and out of prison several times, and the woman from the courts had dealt with her repeatedly. At the same time, scholars (and Sherri) would argue that there was something bigger going on in the woman's hopeless prediction. Assata Zerai and Rae Banks (2002) note:

> Addiction is assumed to lie in the nature of poor Black women. That they perform sex for drugs is taken as proof that they are demons. That they appear not to care about their own health is taken as evidence that they are not human. . . . It is assumed that they do not even care about their children when they engage in behavior that harms them. None of these assumptions takes into account that some poor, under-resourced, disenfranchised, and understandably depressed women with no other options who are suffering from the social disease of addiction engage in the practice of prostitution so that they can afford to dull their pain once again. And these assumptions ignore the reality that lack of access to treatment . . . due to forces beyond their control limits the ability of addicted poor women to protect . . . even their own well-being. (21)

Women in the community believe that dispelling myths about prostitution and drug use is essential to bringing about the broader social and cultural change required to prevent other women from suffering as they have. According to many who live at Magdalene, there is still much work to be done in combating dominant narratives about prostitution, such as the myth that women do not heal. Magdalene residents say that people also believe that women prostitute because it is glamorous or because the women themselves are immoral. During a particularly candid conversation one afternoon at Thistle Farms, Val talked about the images of prostitution she sees in popular culture. She spoke about being on a college campus in Nashville and seeing a sign advertising a sorority and fraternity party with the theme of "Pimps and Hos." "They have *no* idea," she said.

She went on to talk about her belief that most people who have never prostituted romanticize the idea of exchanging sex for money, and that events such as this encourage it. Another woman participating in the conversation said she thought "most people" think women who prostitute do it because they "just really like sex," rather than because "there's a deeper issue." By noting these conflicts, women at Magdalene illustrate some of the representational issues around sex work and those involved. According to Maggie O'Neill (2001), the history of prostitution "is framed by attempts to repress and make morally reprehensible the women involved in prostitution, while aestheticizing the desires and fantasies symbolically associated with the whore, the prostitute, the fallen woman" (129). Thus we see a trend that continues today: one in which the institution of prostitution is frequently divorced from the woman herself, and women's experiences are manipulated to fit available models of acceptable (or unacceptable) sexuality (Nussbaum 1999). In addition to feeling misrepresented by popular symbols of prostitution, the women I interviewed talked about fighting internal battles to uproot such narratives embedded in their notions of the self. I often heard women say things such as, "It has taken me a long time to believe that my body is mine, and I get to decide what happens to it" and "I have to remind myself that I don't have to be in pain — emotionally or physically."

Perhaps no one is as outspoken about prostitution as Becca, and her anger and conviction about the issue are palpable when she speaks:

> I want people to not buy into the myths that are out there in the media about women walking the streets, and that includes things like, "Prostitution is always there" [and] "It's the oldest profession in the world, so it will always be there." And you know, there's no guilt because that's "just how it is," and that's horrible. But when people change their mind culturally, you can really change what the norm is and what's acceptable. You know, we decided that we didn't think

there should be child labor. So we passed these child labor laws and so now, in the US at least, nobody would go around saying like, "Oh, I hire a bunch of kids. They do all my farming, and I can do it all for a dollar an hour." People would be like, "Well, you're screwed up. What is wrong with you?" And so, around this same issue of buying and selling women, *even* if women are willing to be bought and sold, *even* if there are women on the streets who for ten dollars' worth of crack cocaine are willing to get down on their hands and knees and get you off, you would think it's reprehensible to do that to another human being—to use them for your own gain. It's just not acceptable behavior to buy and sell other people. I'm not talking about being judgmental toward the women, I'm talking about that people are willing to buy and sell other people. . . . What we do to women on the Internet, on the street corners, in the jails—it's just universally doing violence on women's bodies. And if you're walking the streets, you're having violence done to your body.

With this statement, Becca is referencing a broader debate that has been around for centuries and exists throughout the world. Discussions about the practice of exchanging sex for money contain a variety of perspectives, including the views of those who say that women who prostitute are themselves immoral, those who argue that the conditions that lead a woman to prostitute are immoral, and those who believe that sex work has nothing to do with morality, but is instead a legitimate way for a woman to use her body to earn a living. Debates about the legality of prostitution correspond to these perspectives, and it seems that there are no easy answers.

Like myths about prostitution, images of drug users can create contexts in which drug use and abuse is synonymous with criminality and deviance. According to the anthropologist Merrill Singer, when it comes to drug users who are also poor, these associations serve the function of providing scapegoats on which to pin social ills generated by structures of inequality. Singer (2008) argues that such users are portrayed as "the social embodiment of nightmarish evil and unlimited harm, and as threats to but not members of society. In other words, drug users serve an important social function as objects of blame: they, not structures of inequality in employment, housing, education, and ownership, are responsible for the social ills that plague everyday life" (232).

The women who speak on behalf of Magdalene work to combat these stereotypes, and do so by sharing their own experiences with the nature of addiction, the difficulty of finding appropriate treatment, and the many material and relational supports required to heal. This message is important, say Magdalene staff members, because the resources for women in recovery are scarce. Becca explained: "There's . . . the myth that there's enough beds out there for women. And I think people think, 'Oh, if you want to get better, you can just go into recovery.' But that's not true. We have women from eight states in the program right now, and women begging *every day* to get in. We have more women wanting to get into the program than we could ever serve."

Like the people who wander into Thistle Farms because they have been encouraged by the stories the women tell, program directors and community members from other programs and communities have begun to come to Magdalene to learn how to respond to the needs and injustices Becca and the women describe when they speak. I was able to interview women from two such communities, and wanted to know: What about Magdalene did they find compelling? What did they learn from hearing the women speak? From visiting? And how was that shaping what they were doing in their own communities?

One woman I interviewed, Susan, was a member of a large church in Atlanta where Becca, Minda, and Kathleen had been to speak. Fascinated by the emphasis on love and grace and the centrality of community in the stories they heard, Susan and other members of her church were compelled to ask themselves, "What's our part in this?" They decided that the first thing they could do was to support Magdalene by selling Thistle Farms products between church services four times a year. A few members of the church then visited Magdalene to learn about replicating the program in Atlanta. Susan reported that one of the most encouraging parts of their trip was that the people she spoke with at Magdalene "were clear that this isn't going to be cookie cutter. Our program isn't going to look like Magdalene, or doesn't have to. Our program can and should respond to the needs and strengths and ways things work in our own community." As a result of their trip, Susan and her friends are in the process of looking for "visionaries" or existing programs in their city that they can support. She said they plan to start small, but it was easy to tell that their dreams and hopes are big.

Julie, whom I mentioned in Chapter 1, is involved with CATCH court in Columbus, Ohio. CATCH (Changing Actions To Change Habits) court is a special program facilitated by the Columbus municipal court system. It serves women who are in court for drugs and prostitution: a judge started the program because he was tired of sentencing the same women to jail or prison, only for them to be back on the streets (and ultimately back in his courtroom) just a few months or years later. The CATCH program allows women to avoid going to jail or prison if they agree to come to court one day a week, participate in outpatient treatment, take drug screens, and complete other requirements such as job training and community service (depending on the nature of their sentence).

Julie is an attorney who runs her own international human rights and anti-trafficking agency. When she decided to get involved with local anti-trafficking efforts, she went to CATCH court to learn about its work. During her first visit, a large group of women was sitting in front of the judge, and he began asking questions: How many of the women had every met their fathers? Two raised their hands. How many of the women had been abandoned by their mothers before age five? Eighty percent raised their hands. How many women had custody of their own children? Not one woman raised her hand.

The women frequenting the municipal court in Columbus were similar to the women I know from Magdalene, and, Julie claims, to women all over the world. Like the staff at Magdalene, Julie and the folks at the court realize that some women are not ready to come off the streets. For the ones who are, however, creating opportunities to leave requires efforts on the part of the entire community. When Julie started working with the court, CATCH had already put many of the community pieces in place, focusing on fostering social connectedness and introducing women to formal and informal resources. For the women in the program, having friends who were sober was at least as important as having access to therapy, and field trips to different community organizations and resources were allowed to replace court dates once a month.

Julie and her agency committed to doing two things to assist CATCH court: coordinate volunteers and coordinate resources. From those duties grew "Bloom!," a formal program serving women with criminal histories that resulted from drug and prostitution charges. Bloom! owns one house (which it operates without live-in authority, thanks to conversations with staff and residents from Magdalene), and has recently begun its own social enterprise: a food cart (cleverly named "Freedom a la Cart") from which Bloom! participants make and sell savory goodies such as empanadas and sandwiches.

Like Thistle Farms, Freedom a la Cart creates a platform from which women from Bloom! can speak out about addiction and prostitution. It also allows women to connect to their communities in such a way that the communities themselves gain a better understanding of experiences—namely addiction, prostitution, and life on the streets— about which they might have only prejudices and stereotypes. And this, says Becca, is the ultimate reason she and Magdalene women spend so much time speaking: the message of Magdalene creates a bridge between women who have been cast aside by their communities and their society, and the communities and social order that cast them aside.

> When we go out there and talk and share things, people are
> humanized for other people. People that may have been written
> off in one sense, or judged so harshly in another sense. You know,
> people say things like, "They just want to be out there, they just want
> to do all that. . . ." No. It's a lot more complicated. And so we're out
> there talking to that same community and reminding them to not be
> judgmental in how they love people. So, that's the wider thing we're
> out there doing.

Narrative theorists alert us, however, that sharing stories with the purpose of creating individual and social change is more than a gesture of reminding or reeducating—it is about *re-creating* the world through language. For example, the work of Nancy Hirschmann draws attention to the relationship between context and the self, particularly as they are both created by and through discourse. This happens on three levels, all of which interact with and rely on each other. The first level, which Hirschmann calls "the ideological representation of reality," is reminiscent of Marx and points to the ways in which language works to create a version of reality that is distorted or incongruent with what is actually occurring. To illustrate this level, Hirschmann provides a litany of "caricatures" that are often used to represent women (e.g., the virgin, the whore, the asexual mother, the sexual temptress) and notes that the problem with these images is that they "fail to recognize women's humanity, their membership in society, their differences from each other, and not just from men, their individuality and their commonality" (78). At the second level of social construction, which Hirschmann calls "materalization," the ideological representation of reality goes beyond distortion and begins to shape the world according to its images. Reality is actually produced by language.[1] At this level, Hirschmann says, "the construction of social behaviors and rules takes on a life of its own, and becomes constitutive not only of what women are allowed to do, but of what they are allowed to be" (79). Environments that constrain and limit some people more than others are created by the ideological beliefs that those persons should be more confined for reasons of desert, protection, or inability. At the third level of social construction, meaning takes its root in language, where it "establishes the parameters for understanding, defining, and communicating about reality, about who women are, what we are doing, what we desire" (80).

Extending these ideas to the Magdalene community demonstrates how the beliefs and narratives against which women in the community are speaking are narratives that influence the very structure of our society and produce women on whom violence and oppression may be exacted. For this reason, combating myths and claiming new narratives is essential for the practice and maintenance of healing, because healing is more than undoing the violence and suffering that one has experienced (Kleinman, Das, and Lock 1997; Das 2001; Hirschmann 2003). It is rather to take the experiences and narratives of violence and suffering (as well as experiences of edification and flourishing) and weave them into new experiences and narratives that allow for and create a new self and subjectivity. For the women at Magdalene, the transformation of personal narratives is an integral part of the healing process, and the public performance of personal narratives that have been transformed through the practice of healing community works to strengthen personal and community narratives, even as they challenge myths and misconceptions.

Contesting Storytelling

Despite the power of oppressive discourses and the need to change them, the work of producing and distributing new narratives poses a variety of conundrums. For example, Becca's stance on prostitution would likely meet with opposition from a variety of groups, not the least from people who point out that the violence often linked with prostitution may be manufactured by the environments in which it takes place (rather than the act itself) (Chapkis 1997; Nagle 1997; Vanwesenbeeck 2001), and those who point out that we *do*, in fact, buy and sell human bodies all the time for a number of different legal and illegal purposes (Bureau of Public Affairs 2010). Furthermore, there is significant evidence that many women who perform sex work deeply resent the idea of one voice speaking for the complexity of experiences subsumed in the practice of "prostitution." For example, a sex worker interviewed by Wendy Chapkis (1997) claimed, "Maybe what they (pro–sex work activists) were doing was glamorous. But they acted like their experience spoke for us all. Well, for the people in my group, it was not glamour" (127). The woman went on to say, however, that anti-prostitution activists also used sex workers as a trope to support their activism more than to help women who were being exploited: "There are others who say that prostitution is evil because it contributes to violence against women and they'll have their 'Take Back the Night' marches right through the Red Light district without even dealing with the sex workers as other women. . . . They just turn us into symbols" (127).

Along these lines, there were a handful of women and staff members I interviewed who were less enthusiastic than Kathleen, Kayla, and others about sharing their stories in public. Although most members of the community saw it as a way to perform new identities and confront negative and pathologizing narratives about addiction and prostitution, others saw telling their stories publicly as exploitative and objectifying. It seemed that the vision of healing the self and others was not intoxicating enough to subdue the realities of addiction and prostitution as experienced by the women at Magdalene, nor was it enough to hide the prejudices of those sitting in the audience. Shelly, a resident who had recently begun speaking at events and home parties, said:

> Sometimes, I feel like I'm being put on display. Some things that have happened to me in my life, I don't really choose to rehash, you know? Sometimes, I honestly feel like when we have some people come and they're like, in awe, like, "This happened?" . . . They're like, "Oh my goodness. You did this, and you did that, and that happened. Oh my God. " And you know, sometimes it makes me feel like I'm being put on a display, you know? 'Cause there are not a whole lot of nice things that we've been through. Being in drug addiction and out on the streets—there's not a whole lot of nice things. And I just don't want to be made to feel like I'm put on display. Period. That's my thing. That's what I think.

Lynn, a Magdalene staff member, goes even further in her criticism of the practice of public storytelling, saying, "It has always concerned me on a number of different levels. I think it's mildly to moderately to even more exploitative of the women. I think it can set certain women up for relapse. You know, everybody can talk a good game, but it's never been clear to me how they feel about it individually. And it's great to, you know, 'gotta talk about it, gotta disclose' . . . but nobody in the audience has to talk about it."

To be clear, no one within Magdalene is ever forced to speak, either privately or publicly, when they do not want to. Speaking has been normalized as a community practice, however, and there are those who believe that this normalcy should be challenged. Marjorie, a Magdalene resident, stated that she didn't mind telling her story, but thought that it should be a practice in which everyone engaged, illustrating the problematic nature of who speaks and why in the context of Magdalene. Speaking to me as a researcher and a volunteer—someone who does not tell my story on a regular basis—Marjorie said:

> I feel like everybody past the age of twenty has a story. And I just think that we shouldn't be the only ones telling our stories. 'Cause I'd like to hear y'all stories, too. 'Cause I know y'all got some. And some of are good, some of 'em may not be good, you know whatever, but I feel like you all should feel just as—I mean the same way you want us to tell our stories, I feel like you all should feel the same way about telling yours. It shouldn't be such a private thing, you know, because the things that we have been through, some of those things have been crucial to us, you know, and detrimental to our life. And so, I mean, that would make me, myself, that would make me feel a lot more comfortable telling my story if we got to hear some of you all's stories, too. 'Cause I feel like everybody in the world's got a story, past the age of twenty-one, whether it's good or bad.

For people who work on issues of voice and power as they relate to justice and well-being, the traditional concern is that some voices have been silenced, and that their silencing is a form of oppression (Das 2001). In this case, it appears that the opposite is true—that there are times when amplifying the voices of those who have been silenced can be destructive as well, particularly when the amplified voices work to reify divisions that exist between people based on life experiences that have been shaped by injustice.

Getting There

The conversation with Marjorie in which she asked why I never had to tell my story took place in the context of a focus group. I had asked a group of Magdalene residents and graduates specifically about their experiences with "telling their story" to public audiences (or to me, a researcher). After Marjorie's comment, I asked her, somewhat uncertainly, "Do you want me to tell you 'my story'?" She nodded, and

I said, "Right now?" She and others in the group nodded again. After spending months in the community interviewing and observing
people, I felt that honoring their request was the appropriate thing to
do. I told my story, being careful to include details with which they
might connect and which I thought would confirm Marjorie's suspi-
cion that I, too, must have a story: details about addiction and recovery
in my own family, details about times when I had felt alone or afraid or
cast out, details about times when I had felt loved and valued and included, details about my own experiences with God, and details about
other events that have come to define me. After what felt like a long
and uncomfortably intimate disclosure, I stopped talking. Not leaving
any room for silence, Marjorie said, "That's it?"

I was not exactly sure how to respond to someone who had just implied that my life was charmed and its story boring to the point of being disappointing, so I said, "Well, it's not selling any Thistle Farms
products." Everyone in the focus group laughed, and we went on with
the rest of the discussion, but the moment had been profound, as were
Marjorie's words. Based on my experience at Magdalene and in life in
general, I believe that there is deep and healing truth to the idea that,
as Minda told me at the copy machine, "we're all broken and we all
need each other"—truth to the idea that when a community of people
comes together, we all have wounds and scars, regardless of life experience. On the other hand, there is also truth in recognizing differences.
It does not make the world or even the community of Magdalene a
more just place if everyone pretends that all the scars and wounds are
the same. There is truth in recognizing that I have never spent even
one night on the streets, that I have never been thrown over a balcony
railing, never been shot, never been beaten, never been abused, and
that my family has never been so marginalized that I would need to sell
my body to help my mother pay our bills. There is also truth in recognizing that many of the women at Magdalene fight harder every day to
stay clean than I have ever fought for anything. The problem, it seems,
comes when life experiences and identity narratives define us beyond
the ability to move past them, or when they are used to flatten the tex-
tures of human experience in an effort to make them fit categories of

"good" and "bad." Thomas, a volunteer and board member who has been involved with the community since its formation, noted this tension: They deserve the spotlight, you know. They deserve to stand up and tell the world, "Look at me. I was that way, and I'm now this way." But, you know, I think that that's not the end of their journey. Marion can go and tell that story, but she doesn't tell that story anymore. Her whole life doesn't have to be defined by her recovery, by her prostitution that's now been reversed."

Thomas added that a next step for Magdalene would be figuring out how to free the women from being defined by their lives on the street. Pondering phrases such as "I am Marion, a recovering prostitute," he asked, "Why do you even have to have that anymore? Can't you go on and just talk about, 'I am Marion, the mother of so and so, and I'm this and I'm that, and I'm that.' . . . But I don't know how you get there."

The challenge of "getting there" is an important one, and one that has serious implications for promoting human flourishing. As we shall see in the next chapter, moving past experiences with addiction and prostitution is difficult, even for the most "successful" Magdalene graduates. Tremendous physical, psychological, and spiritual healing occurs for many, many women who walk through the Magdalene community, and this healing results in greater freedom to make desired choices, to be one's self, and to participate in relationships that support rather than restrict human flourishing. However, when the women of Magdalene leave the community to seek out life on their own, they often find their healed selves confronting an unhealed outside world that makes basic necessities such as staying clean, finding a job, and maintaining housing incredibly difficult.

CHAPTER 8

Healing Still

I give them credit for saving my life—or, actually, giving
me life. Because I didn't really have a life, you know?
Unless you consider walking up and down the streets,
selling your body for your next hit "having a life." But
once I was willing to get some help, to do something
different, and once I was able to forgive myself and other
people, I was able to heal. I was able to stop holding all
that resentment and that anger and that animosity. I was
able to live.

—Sherri, Magdalene House graduate

W<small>HEN WOMEN COMPARE THEIR</small> lives before Magdalene to
their lives during and after, they draw stark contrasts that indicate the powerful change in both their circumstances and their notions
of self. They talk about the transitions they experienced using phrases
such as "going from darkness to light," "fear to courage," "bondage to
freedom," "scarcity to abundance," and "death to life." It is because of
these kinds of transitions—and the power to be able to proclaim them
in private rooms and public spaces alike—that Becca Stevens named
the community "Magdalene": according to all four Gospels in the
Christian Bible, Mary Magdalene was the first person to see the risen
Christ and to tell others about his resurrection from the dead. Community members say that Magdalene House is named after this iconic
woman not because of her association with prostitution (which is more

speculation and tradition than substantive claim; see Carroll 2009), but because she was the first preacher of the resurrection.

Just as the resurrection is understood to be miraculous by those within the Christian faith, the changes that occur for women at Magdalene are understood to be the work of something divine. Whether women describe the divine as "God," "my higher power," or any other name (e.g., "Love," "Grace," "Truth"), it is evident that the hospitality and healing they experience within the Magdalene community marks Magdalene House as sacred space. Furthermore, according to the women at Magdalene, "Love" is both the method and the reason for healing—love for self, for their friends and families, for their children, and for each other—the kind of love that says, "You're valuable and beautiful in your brokenness" and "I love you, come as you are."

I sat in on a writing class during which women from Magdalene worked with a local author to write poetry about their experiences. The women wrote about their families and the streets, as well as about their newfound home and the love they had found there. They described love as "open arms," "the opposite of judgment," "something that makes you whole," "intense affection," and "a yes." They characterized it as unending and unconditional—something that saw goodness and potential in even the bleakest of stories. I know from listening to Becca that her vision of God and the world in which we live is that nothing is left to be condemned—that there is opportunity for wholeness, worth, and belonging for all things, and that love and mercy are the source and practice of being made whole.

Of the women I interviewed who had been through the Magdalene program, eleven of nineteen said, unprompted, that they had believed they would die on the streets, and credit Magdalene for their being alive today. Kathleen had begged God to let her die or send her to jail (see Chapter 2), but "thanks to God and to Magdalene," she got off the streets, got clean, and now helps other women recover from addiction. Describing how she began to talk to God, Kathleen said: "I can remember looking at the crack pipe and telling myself, 'I know what you're all about.' And I remember looking up at the sky, and saying, 'OK, God, I'm fixin' to step out on faith. I don't have a clue where you're going to take me, but I'm fixin' to walk.' So I got in that [police] car, put my head down, and asked them to drive off."

Kathleen's journey toward recovery started with a prayer, and when she tells her story, images of transformation encompass both the growing importance of God in her life and her own experiences of conquering addiction and escaping death on the streets. Other women who survived the streets by stealing and exacting violence on others report that healing from addiction allows them to "be somebody different today." As the women tell it, being "somebody different" means being honest, trustworthy, and responsible—doing things of which they are proud. Gloria told me that one of the biggest changes in her life since she entered Magdalene House is that she has stopped stealing, even though it sometimes still requires concentrated effort:

> I've been out there on the street for damn near forty-five years, and this is all I know. I got that street mentality—the lying, the stealing, everything, the manipulation, all of that. Before, I called myself one of the best boosters there was. I ain't boost out of no bag—I wore a girdle. And I came back like I had a big bag, you know what I'm saying? I would go into them stores and take people's stuff like it was mine. I paid my way, and I don't know how many others way. Every day. [But] I'm able to recognize today. I don't go into a store and don't pick up nothin'—ain't nothin' but five cents, I'm going to pay for it. I'm able to be honest today—I don't care how bad it hurt.

The idea that people are changed in and through loving relationships applies to more than the women who come to Magdalene as residents—it applies to volunteers, staff members, and visitors as well. If the statement that "we're all broken and we all need each other" holds true, then participation in the Magdalene community should bring about transformation in the lives of the people who support Magdalene. Jenny, a full-time volunteer at Thistle Farms, told me that Magdalene has helped her see the many things in her life she had taken for granted, and talked about how her experiences in the community have helped pave the way for a life filled with gratitude. She went on to say,

"Many of us wouldn't be living the lives that we are living if it wasn't for Magdalene. And it has given me—it has given my life a new perspective. I feel like I'm fulfilling a purpose."

Andrea, a former staff member at Thistle Farms, told me about a specific instance in which the Magdalene community helped her to see her own prejudices:

> One of the moments that really stands out for me is one of the first times I took a group to a bank. There was gonna be a holiday party, so this was probably like around Christmas when I had started working in September, and we were going to set up and sell in this bank. And after we were done, there were three women, and we were all packed in my car, and we started driving, and all three of those women pulled out their cell phones and called their children. And I remember being surprised by that, and then feeling sort of a little bit chagrined. . . . Because I hadn't seen them with their children, I hadn't thought of them in terms of being mothers. And that was an expansion of my idea of a prostitute or a drug addict. . . . It was sort of like, "Oh, and they have children." And the fact that they were asking their kids about their homework really struck me.

Bringing people together in a community context does more than help women get off the streets. It allows people to examine their own lives and beliefs, and the way these things affect others. During my time at Magdalene, I saw people from all walks of life come together, relate to one another, and work toward common purposes. I watched a woman who lives in Al Gore's upper-class Nashville neighborhood learn to make candles from a woman whose inconvenient truth is that she once turned a trick to pay her electric bill. While Magdalene is certainly not immune to the invisibility of privilege that exists throughout the world, it provides a context in which relationships and experiences such as these can occur—relationships and experiences that have the *potential* to uncover privilege and challenge oppression.

Beyond the Magdalene Community:
Barriers to Living Free

Those within the Magdalene community argue that recovery would be easier if relationships such as those described here happened more often. Much like Mary Magdalene, women who preach resurrection are often met with doubt and skepticism from those outside the Magdalene community. Furthermore, they often find that the exercise of a "reformed" self is made difficult by the "unreformed" world they reenter (Snarr 2007). Although the audiences who gather to hear the women tell their stories are almost always receptive and appreciative, prior interactions and criminal histories often speak louder than claims of reform when it comes to family members, landlords, and potential employers. Sadly, when women leave Magdalene, they are confronted by communities and systems that neither acknowledge their hard-won accomplishments nor alleviate their struggles (Kelly 2006; Snarr 2007). Among other things, this makes the challenges of staying clean, securing housing, and finding employment all the more profound.

STAYING CLEAN
When women begin to transition out of Magdalene, staying clean is of utmost importance to them, as well as to the staff. When I interviewed her, Natalie was staying in one of Magdalene's transition houses but preparing to live on her own sometime within the next few months. She described her experience:

> Being out of the program and kind of being on my own, I can say that it's not easy to stay clean, but it's not hard either, because I know what I want. I know that I don't want to be in that lifestyle anymore. But I do have to do the work. I go to meetings, and I try to keep myself surrounded with the women. I try to keep myself around people who don't do drugs and aren't in that lifestyle. And that makes it pretty easy for me to stay clean. I am scared about when I get my own place and stuff and I won't be around the women as much as I have been. You know, it does make me nervous, but like I said, I know what I want. I

know I don't want to use, and I know what I have to do to stay clean. As long as I continue to take those steps, I have a bright future.

Connection to a supportive community and to other people in recovery is a tested strategy for staying clean (Gossop, Stewart, and Marsden 2007), as is maintaining goals for the future. For the women in the Magdalene program with young children, regaining custody is often their most motivating goal. When I asked Natalie what she wanted for herself in the future, she said:

> I would have custody back of my son. I would have a nice place to live—you know, somewhere safe and secure for me and him, and really, just kind of doing the same thing I'm doing. I like working for Thistle Farms. I can't say that I'm gonna stay there forever, 'cause I don't know, but I would say I'll be working for Thistle Farms, and being able to provide for me and my son. That would be a dream come true for me.

It would seem that dreams as simple as having a safe place to live, an enjoyable place to work, and a healthy relationship with one's child would be easy to come by—such desires reflect human capabilities at their most basic level (Nussbaum 2000). Reality, however, is not always simple, particularly for women leaving Magdalene. For some, two years has not been long enough to heal from a lifetime of abuse and the trauma of living on the streets. For others, the poor work histories and criminal records they accumulated while they were in active addiction are difficult to escape, despite the adequate job skills and positive recommendations they have obtained in the course of their recovery. Contrasting the prospects of Magdalene graduates with those of others, a Magdalene staff member said, "I do think it has a lot to do with socioeconomic status." She asserted that people from middle- and upper-income backgrounds who are addicted "can get into recovery, they get clean, and because they have some of that other support in their life, . . . they can go on and live fairly stable lives." By contrast, she lamented that "getting the women [at Magdalene] clean from alcohol and drug use doesn't necessarily prevent them from relapsing and it surely doesn't guarantee that they aren't going to continue to have a good bit of trouble in life."

This assessment of the socioeconomic factors in maintaining sobriety points to the interlocking nature of various types of injustice (and poor health) (Farmer 1999; Snarr 2007). It also illustrates once again the variability of consequences for those who experience addiction (Roberts, Jackson, and Carlton-LaNey 2000).

FINDING EMPLOYMENT

Perhaps because I spent so much time at Thistle Farms, and many of the women who work there aspire to move on to new and different jobs, I was struck by how the challenge of finding a job seemed to be a constant struggle. Natalie, a Magdalene graduate who has a high school diploma and excellent work skills, recently looked for work to subsidize her part-time position as the office manager of Thistle Farms. Before coming to Magdalene, Natalie spent six months on the streets (much less time than most Magdalene residents and graduates), during which she acquired several misdemeanor charges: indecent exposure, theft of gasoline, possession of cocaine, soliciting prostitution, and assault. Although Natalie has been clean, housed, employed, and violation free for three years, she was turned down for most jobs. During one particularly embarrassing incident, Natalie was hired to work at McDonald's and then fired in the middle of a training session. On her first day of work, she was sitting with other trainees in the back room, watching a video about food preparation, when the manager came in and pulled her aside. Apparently, the manager had not run her background check during the hiring process, and ran it instead while she was completing her training. Once he saw her record, he realized his "mistake" (according to McDonald's policy) and worked quickly to undo it. He abruptly handed Natalie a printout of her record, said, "You can't work here," and pushed her toward the door. Natalie did eventually find a job at an ice cream shop, and works there part time in addition to Thistle Farms.

When I asked the women I interviewed what they wanted to do once they got back on their feet, their aspirations were varied: Mattie wanted to go to school to become a beautician, Sasha wanted to start her own in-home catering business, Mary was interested in working with computers, and Paula was enrolled in college classes to obtain her prerequisites for nursing school. Paula's road had not been easy: she came to Magdalene with prior student loan debt and thousands of dollars of unpaid taxes. Her first year at Magdalene, everything she earned at Thistle Farms went to pay her creditors, and Magdalene matched her efforts. Becca described the philosophy behind the Individual Development Account (IDA) program, saying that it was designed to free the women from debt so they don't have to go back into the world fighting an uphill battle:

> The reason that we started the IDA accounts and to match the women's money they save was so, if you're saving $1,000, it takes you forever, but the incentive should double it, and that means that if you can put $2,000 down on a car, that one car, that starter car, is not going to strap you in for five years and that you never get ahead. I mean, part of the thing of poverty is that you never get ahead, so you're always pushing from behind. And there is no freedom in doing that. So my thing is that if you stay for two years and you really save and we double your savings or whatever, that you can make a dent and get ahead a little bit.

This strategy worked for Paula, who was able to start attending classes at a local community college during her second year at Magdalene. At the time of my research, Paula was working part time at Thistle Farms, going to school, and living in a house given to her by a member of her church. Describing her long-term plans, Paula said:

> What I really want to do with this degree is to do some home health care for the elderly because I realize that not only are there problems with homeless people and the drug addicted and the mentally ill, there also are problems with the elderly. And that's my goal right now. . . . I'm fifty-three, and I probably won't graduate from school until I am fifty-seven. [*laughs*] But I'm determined to do this, and I'm determined to do the best that I can. Last semester was a bit of

a challenge—I ended up with Cs in both classes. . . . I didn't have the availability, the access [to a computer]. But now I have my own computer, my own printer, I'm online, and that's huge. Because I spent a tremendous amount of time in the library last semester, and, you know, where now I can get way ahead of myself like on all of my papers, and save them and come back to them, and so now I've got stuff ready that's not even due until April.

According to research on physical and mental health as well as studies of general well-being, the ability to work in a job that is safe, fulfilling, and justly compensated is an essential component of human flourishing (Fryer and Fagan 2003). However, the stories of Paula, Natalie, and others like them demonstrate that finding such employment is often the exception instead of the rule (Hartmann 2003; Hardaway and McLoyd 2009). Furthermore, their experiences highlight many of the mechanisms (both formal and informal) that keep people marginalized regardless of skill, ability, or special circumstance (Farmer 1999; James et al. 2003; Kelly 2006). For many people, at Magdalene and elsewhere, the freedom to work and the right to work with dignity are undermined by an economic system in which employees are valued as little more than cogs in a machine (Folbre et al. 1992). Thistle Farms' commitment to providing employment to women from Magdalene regardless of skill or ability posits a radically different economic form. Similar organizations—such as Greyston Bakery in Yonkers, New York, whose mission statement reads, "We don't hire people to bake brownies. We bake brownies to hire people" (*www.greystonbakery.com*)—demonstrate that alternative business models can succeed (Gibson-Graham 2006). Still, the challenges of staying financially solvent and continuing to employ the women for whom Thistle Farms exists require a tremendous balancing act in which Becca, Holli, and the managing council must try to integrate noncapitalist commitments with a capitalist market.

For the most part, women who leave Magdalene and find employment remain among the working poor. Many continue to work in highly gendered professions such as professional caregiving and housekeeping, which tend to be less secure as well as disproportionately underpaid (Estévez-Abe 2006). These jobs are, of course, essential to a functioning society. The important point at this juncture is not so much whether these jobs should be marginalized (I believe they should not), but rather that they *are*. Like many other Nashville residents who earn below a living wage, the women who leave Magdalene find it difficult, if not impossible, to maintain essentials for living such as housing, transportation, food, and health care. Additionally, the stress of living such an economically marginal existence can threaten the mental and physical health of women fighting to recover (Kasper et al. 2008). In these cases, women are sometimes tempted to return to selling drugs because it is a lucrative and easy practice, not to mention the status it had provided to them on the streets. Interestingly, in my two years at Magdalene, I never heard a woman say she wanted to return to prostitution, even though several feminist theorists note that there are many similarities between prostitution and other gendered, low-paying, or physically demanding forms of work (Chapkis 1997; Nagle 1997; Nussbaum 2000).

SECURING HOUSING

Obtaining a safe and affordable place to live upon leaving Magdalene is paramount to maintaining recovery, and the stress of finding such housing is palpable among women reaching the end of their two years in the program. Magdalene has been able to assist many of its graduates by providing transitional housing and by helping graduates purchase their own homes. As of 2009, the transition home houses three graduates at a time, and each woman pays one hundred dollars a month for rent, plus one-third of the utilities. Ideally, a woman lives in the transition home for a year, during which she establishes better credit and practices budgeting money, as well as continuing to save to be on her own. In the first two years of Magdalene's transitional housing initiative, five women lived in the transition home, some for only a few months, some for over a year. Kayla and Stacia, two graduates who purchased their own homes with the help of Magdalene, did so through a federal buy-down grant that allowed Magdalene to cosign the mortgages and enabled the women to build their own houses for much less than the market value. The security and accomplishment of owning one's own home are a source of great pride for Kayla and Stacia, as well as for the entire Magdalene community.

There is high hope in the community that similar opportunities will be afforded to other graduates, although Mindy and Stacia were "best-case scenarios"—neither had felonies on her record, both had stable jobs, and both had long-term partners to help with the mortgage and utilities. For women who have more extensive criminal records or are on their own financially, finding a place to live often seems a near impossibility. Michelle, a Magdalene graduate who has been clean, steadily employed, and violation free for eight years, recently divorced her husband and began looking for an apartment for herself and her fifteen-year-old daughter. Michelle's experience with apartment hunting has not been unlike Natalie's experience looking for a job. At one place she applied, the manager refused to rent to her after doing a background check, and told her never to return to the premises. Michelle admits that her record is "impressive," but also asks, "Haven't I proven otherwise?" To date, Michelle is still looking for a place to live, and says she feels her options are limited—the places that she can afford and that will take her with her record are not places where she wants to live or to raise her daughter.

Again, the experiences of Michelle and women like her are more than just stories of individual suffering and frustration. Their difficulty in securing safe and affordable housing is indicative of larger trends in the Nashville housing market. According to the Tennessee Housing Development Agency (2009), the hourly wage needed to buy a house at the median home price in Davidson County in 2008 was $25.26, and $21.17 in the state of Tennessee. The hourly wage needed to rent a two-bedroom apartment at the median rental price in 2008 was $11.61 in Davidson County, and $12.38 in the state of Tennessee overall. Given that the minimum wage was $6.55, these prices meant that many people who worked full-time jobs could not rent an apartment or buy a house at the median price.

While there are, of course, cheaper houses and apartments available, often these places come with poorly performing schools, higher crime rates (Galster and Santiago 2006), and decreased access to neighborhood resources (Kuno and Rothbard 2005). Women who cannot secure or maintain housing often end up living with siblings, cousins, or partners. While this is sometimes a good option, it often leads to their living in environments they have neither the power to control nor the resources to exit.

Despite the stories of continued struggle, it is important to emphasize that the women who come through Magdalene and are able to get clean, access necessary services, create healthy identities, and experience positive relationships would be the first to insist that their lives today are better than they were before. According to these women, living in an apartment or with relatives is preferable to living on the streets any day, and earning money at a restaurant is a tremendous victory compared with turning tricks on Dickerson Road. Furthermore, staff and volunteers at Magdalene experience healing from being in a community that allows them to examine their own prejudices and brokenness and to seek support through loving relationships. Residents, graduates, staff, and volunteers alike talk about the healing Magdalene House makes possible by being a community committed to truth-telling and acceptance. Still, there is more work to be done, and the changes made within the community are only lasting to the extent that other, healthy communities and systems are developed (Prilleltensky and Nelson 2002).

Some psychologists make a clear distinction between "ameliorative change" and "transformative change." Ameliorative change works largely to teach individuals to function within current economic, social, and political systems, whereas transformative change works to change oppressive systems of injustice in the belief that individual-level change will follow (Bess et al. 2009). An example of ameliorative change would be teaching women job skills so they can climb the economic ladder, a positive change for the women involved. However, this does not provide an answer for the women unable to work themselves up the economic ladder or the millions of persons working minimum-wage jobs, nor does it answer how those jobs are going to be accomplished in the event that everyone "works up." A transformative change would be one that allows women to acquire job skills should they so desire them, but also alters wage structures and employment scenarios to provide living wages and benefits to all workers, regardless of type of work.

Changes such as these are changes recommended by theories of structural violence and social suffering, which argue for social institutions that support human capabilities for all (Nussbaum 2000), the re-creation of social and political structures through liberating discourse (Hirschmann 2003), and the centering of care as a vital human activity worthy of political and economic recognition (Kittay 1998, 2001; Tronto 1993). These transformations do not happen without a politically engaged public, however, and political sensibilities develop at the level of relationships and collectivities (Eliasoph 1998; Rochon 2000). For this reason, communities and community organizations are prime mechanisms through which to develop individual participation, political aptitude, and critical consciousness that could then used collectively to bring about social change. According to Kimberly Bess et al. (2009), local communities and community organizations have the potential to work toward the goals of "seeking to challenge existing power hierarchies, privileging local knowledge, building on the strengths and gifts each member brings to the table" (12).

At the same time, it seems that many justice-based theories of health and healing rely on a belief that changing social structures alone would lead to human liberation, if only we could make it happen. The work of other theorists, as well as the stories of self provided by the participants in my study, demonstrates that an adequately sophisticated understanding of the self is one in which the self is *created* through narratives, relationships, and systems, as opposed to merely embedded in them. If selves are created through the systems in which they are embedded, changing systems alone will not lead to individual change, nor will systems change occur without individual change and community change—the re-creation of society requires the re-creation of selves, the re-creation of selves requires the re-creation of society, and all is accomplished through and in relationship. In this sense, it seems that the self requires a context in which it can be re-created along with other selves, accompanied by narratives of dignity and belonging.

One of the many privileges of doing this research was the opportunity to talk with men and women who work every day to make the world a better place. They reminded me that while the work of healing is hard, its tenets are simple. In the words of Father Charlie Strobel:

> People always say, "Well, what do the homeless need?" or "What do the women of Magdalene need?" They need what all of us need. They need what *all of us* need. They need the basic necessities of food, clothing, and shelter. They need the second level of social needs — of education and belonging, and a sense of social connection. And then they need those higher needs of having purpose and meaning in life and trying to make sense of it all. And we need those things to make us happy, and they need those things, too. I want to push it a little bit and say that some of those needs are basic human rights. You know, housing and food and clothing and health care and necessary social services. And not to have those things is to live in a subhuman existence.

CONCLUSION

EVERY YEAR AT MAGDALENE House's fundraising benefit, the staff gives the Julia Basquette Award to the "volunteer of the year." The award is named in memory of a former Magdalene resident who left the program to care for her ailing mother, relapsed, and returned to the streets, where she was killed by a trick. In the face of such brutality, the women at Magdalene look at Julia's death and say God was merciful for allowing her to die instead of continuing to endure the hellish life of the streets. To say that the streets were worse than death is not a stretch for many of the women who come to Magdalene. To know that relapse sometimes leads them back is to know something about the power of addiction. To sit in the meditation circle at Thistle Farms when a woman says, "Today is my one-year birthday—I've been clean for 365 days," and hear everyone else shout, whistle, and cheer, is to catch a glimmer of the mystery and miracle of healing.

In his essay "Health as Membership," Wendell Berry writes, "I believe that community—in the fullest sense: a place and all its creatures—is the smallest unit of health and that to speak of the health of an isolated individual is a contradiction in terms." For Berry, who understands health as "wholeness," the practice of healing is one in which the disconnected fragments of self, other, and world are harmoniously reintegrated. Health is more than a lack of illness; it is, as Berry's title states, a practice of belonging. A key premise of this definition is that membership is a condition of health, rather than health acting as a ticket to membership. People don't become healthy and then enter into community; rather, they enter into community to become healthy, and participate in community to maintain health.

Throughout this book, I have used the word "community" because it was a word I heard often at Magdalene, and a word that residents, graduates, staff, and volunteers used to create a meaningful representation of how they experienced their relationships to each other. "Community" implied that their group was more than a collection of individuals, and more than a program or an organization. It meant that they were bound by relationships of care and obligation, and that their identities were, at least in part, constituted by "belonging" at Magdalene. Additionally, women at Magdalene often used the word "community" when calling on others to join their efforts for love and healing. For example, people would say, "The Nashville community should care about X," or "When we speak about Magdalene in public, we're reminding the community to be accepting and nonjudgmental." In these senses, the word "community" was a powerful tool used to imply that there should be relationships of obligation and identification, even if there were not.

At the same time, the word "community" can be troublesome. It creates the illusion of something that is definable and static, which communities almost never are. There seems to be a tendency to view communities as entities that are inherently good when, in fact, many are often quite violent and oppressive. Finally, the work of creating and maintaining community solidarity can eclipse internal injustices and silence dissent. It seems, then, that the qualities of a community are at least as important as the community itself. Health requires membership, but at least for the women at Magdalene, membership means something specific.

Magdalene House's approach to membership—*come as you are*—means that women can come in off the streets without having to shower, clean up their language, or check their cigarettes at the door. It means that they can come in sick, broken, and ragged. They can come in fearful, angry, and desperate. They can come in poor, hungry, and feeling like they have nothing to contribute, because someone in the community believes that they are valuable and worthy of love just as they are. During my interviews, I asked each person, "If you would say that Magdalene as a community has a story, what would it be?" People gave different answers—answers that had to do with love, courage, freedom, provision, and healing. Healing came up most often, and often the message was simple: healing is possible—for all of us. This belief represents a message of hope spoken to everyone who has struggled with addiction and believed it might never end, and to everyone who has loved people who struggle with addiction and believed that their loved ones might never be free. It is a message to people who have broken bodies, unstable minds, or damaged relationships—either by their doing or the doing of others—that illness is acceptable and transformable, and that it does not have to be experienced alone or in shame.

NOTES

INTRODUCTION

1. In this book, pseudonyms have been used for all Magdalene residents, graduates, staff, and volunteers, as well as individuals mentioned in interviews, with the exception of Becca Stevens, Holli Anglin, and Charlie Strobel.
2. In contrast, the total US population increased by only 30 percent during the same period.

CHAPTER 1

1. Twelve-step philosophy is an approach to recovery from addiction that relies on twelve guiding principles, such as "we admitted we were powerless over [object of addiction]—that our lives had become unmanageable," and includes programs such as Alcoholics Anonymous and Narcotics Anonymous.
2. The Prostitution Solicitation School is an eight-hour educational program offered to men who have been arrested as first-time offenders for soliciting prostitutes. As of December 2009, an estimated 3,228 individuals had attended the school per their pre-trial diversion agreements with Nashville's criminal courts.

CHAPTER 2

1. By comparison, the American Academy of Pediatrics estimates that one in twenty US children is physically, sexually, or emotionally abused each year.
2. Kayla used the phrase "friend girl" to indicate a girl who was a friend in the platonic sense. "Girlfriend" indicated a girl with whom one was romantically involved.

CHAPTER 5

1. In general, women who enter Magdalene have children but do not have custody of them at the time they enter, for obvious reasons. Helping residents regain custody of their children (should they so desire it) is one of the program goals of Magdalene; however, this rarely happens until the end of the two-year residency is near, at the earliest.
2. When I presented these findings to the women in the Magdalene community, their loudest complaint was about my categorization of cigarettes as "nonessential."

CHAPTER 7

1. This idea is also borrowed from Marx, who describes how capitalist ideology produces relationships of alienation between workers and other workers, workers and themselves, and workers and their labor.

REFERENCES

Alcoff, L. (1991). The problem of speaking for others. *Cultural Critique* (Winter), 5–32.

Berlin, I. (1971). Two concepts of liberty. In *Four essays on liberty*. New York: Oxford University Press, 118–72.

Berry, W. (1996). *Another turn of the crank*. Washington, DC: Counterpoint.

Bess, K., Prilleltensky, I., Perkins, D., and Collins, L. (2009). Participatory organizational change in community-based health and human services: From tokenism to political engagement. *American Journal of Community Psychology, 43*, 134–48.

Bindel, J., and Kelly, L. (2004). *A critical examination of responses to prostitution in four countries: Victoria, Australia; Ireland; the Netherlands; and Sweden*. London: Child and Women Abuse Studies Unit.

Binswanger, I. A., Stern, M. F., Deyo, R. A., Heagerty, P. J., Cheadle, A., Elmore, J. G., and Koepsell, T. D. (2007). Release from prison—a high risk of death for former inmates. *New England Journal of Medicine, 356,* 157–65.

Bolton, D., Hill, J., O'Ryan, D., Udwin, O., Boyle, S., and Yule, W. (2004). Long-term effects of psychological trauma on psychosocial functioning. *Journal of Child Psychology and Psychiatry, 45*(5), 1007–1014.

Bowden, P. (2006). Embodied care: Jane Addams, Maurice Merleau-Ponty, and feminist ethics. *Hypatia, 21*(3), 210–16.

Boyte, H. (2003). A different kind of politics: John Dewey and the meaning of citizenship in the 21st century. *Good Society, 12*(2), 3–15.

Brady, K., and Back, S. (2009). *Women and addiction: A comprehensive handbook*. New York: Guilford Press.

Brison, S. (2002). Violence and the remaking of a self. *Chronicle of Higher Education, 48*(19).

Bureau of Public Affairs. (2010). *Trafficking in persons: Ten years of partnering to combat modern slavery*. Washington, DC: US Department of State. Retrieved September 24, 2011 from *www.state.gov/r/pa/scp/ fs/2010/143115.htm*.

Carroll, J. (2009). *Practicing Catholic*. New York: Houghton Mifflin Harcourt.

Caughy, M. O., and O'Campo, P. J. (2006). Neighborhood impoverishment, social capital, and the cognitive development of African American pre-schoolers. *American Journal of Community Psychology, 37*(1–2), 141–54.

Chapkis, W. (1997). *Live sex acts: Women performing erotic labor*. New York: Routledge.

Christensen, R., Hodgkins, C., Garces, L., and Estlund, K. (2005). Homeless, mentally ill and addicted: The need for abuse and trauma services. *Journal of Health Care for the Poor and Underserved, 16*(4), 615–22.

Chua, P., Bhavnani, K., and Foran, J. (2000). Women, culture, development: A new paradigm for development studies? *Ethnic and Racial Studies, 23*(5), 820–41.

Coakley, S., and Shelemay, K. (2007). *Pain and its transformations*. Cambridge, MA: Harvard University Press.

Das, V. (2001). *Remaking a world: Violence, social suffering, and recovery*. Berkeley: University of California Press.

Denzin, N., and Lincoln, Y. (2005). *The Sage handbook of qualitative research*. 3rd ed. Thousand Oaks, CA: Sage Publications.

DeVoe, J., Graham, A., Angier, H., Baez, A., and Krois, L. (2008). Obtaining health care services for low-income children: A hierarchy of needs. *Journal of Health Care for the Poor and Underserved, 19*(4), 1192–211.

de Waal, E. (2001). *Seeking God: The way of St. Benedict*. Collegeville, MN: Liturgical Press.

Dilorio, C., Hartwell, T., and Hansen, N. (2002). Childhood sexual abuse and risk behaviors among men at high risk for HIV infection. *American Journal of Public Health, 92*(2), 214–19.

Dunlap, E., Golub, A., Johnston, B., and Wesley, D. (2002). Intergenerational transmission of conduct norms for drugs, sexual exploitation and violence: A case study. *British Journal of Criminology, 42*(1), 1–29.

Durr, M. (2005). Sex, drugs, and HIV: Sisters of Laundromat. *Gender and Society, 19*, 721–28.

Elias, J. (2007). Sex worker union organizing: an international study. *Capital and Class, 93*, 273–76.

Eliasoph, N. (1998). *Avoiding politics: How Americans produce apathy in everyday life*. Cambridge: Cambridge University Press.

Emmons, R. A., and McCullough, M. E. (2004). *The psychology of gratitude*. New York: Oxford University Press.

Estévez-Abe, M. (2006). Gendering the varieties of capitalism: A study of occupational segregation by sex in advances industrial societies. *World Politics*, 59(1), 142–78.

Fadiman, A. (1997). *The spirit catches you and you fall down*. New York: Farrar, Straus and Giroux.

Fals-Borda, O. (1987). The application of participatory action-research in Latin America. *International Sociology*, 2, 329–47.

Fals-Borda, O. (1991). *Action and knowledge: Breaking the monopoly with participatory action research*. New York: Apex Press.

Farley, M., and Barkan, H. (1998). Prostitution, violence, and post-traumatic stress disorder. *Women and Health* 27(3), 37–49

Farmer, P. (1999). *Pathologies of power: Health, human rights, and the new war on the poor*. Berkeley: University of California Press.

Floyd-Thomas, S. (2006). *Mining the motherlode: Methods in womanist ethics*. Cleveland: Pilgrim Press.

Folbre, N., Bergmann, B., Agarwal, B., and Floro, M. (1992). *Women's work in the world economy*. New York: New York University Press.

Foster-Fishman, P., Nowell, B., Deacon, Z., Nievar, M. A., and McCann, P. (2005). Using methods that matter: The impact of reflection, dialogue, and voice. *American Journal of Community Psychology*, 36(3/4), 275–91.

Fryer, D., and Fagan, R. (2003). Poverty and unemployment. In S. C. Carr and T. S. Sloan (Eds.), *Poverty and psychology: From global perspective to local practice*. New York: Kluwer Academic Press. 87–102.

Galster, G. C., and Santiago, A. M. (2006). What's the 'hood got to do with it? Parental perceptions about how neighborhood mechanisms affect their children. *Journal of Urban Affairs*, 28(3), 201–227.

Gebhardt, E. (1982). Introduction to part 3 (A critique of methodology). In A. Arato and E. Gebhardt (Eds.), *The essential Frankfurt School reader*. New York: Continuum. 371–406.

Gibson-Graham, J. K. (2006). *A post-capitalist politics*. Minneapolis: University of Minnesota Press.

Golembeski, C., and Fullilove, R. E. (2005). Criminal (in)justice in the city and its associated health consequences. *American Journal of Public Health*, 95, 1701–6.

Goodyear, M., and Cusick, L. (2007). Protection of sex workers. *British Medical Journal*, 334, 52–53.

Gossop, M., Stewart, D., and Marsden, J. (2007). Attendance at Narcotics Anonymous and Alcoholic Anonymous meetings, frequency of attendance, and substance use outcomes after residential treatment for drug dependence: A 5-year follow-up study. *Addiction*, 103, 119–25.

Hardaway, C., and McLoyd, V. (2009). Escaping poverty and securing middle class status: How race and socioeconomic status shape mobility prospects for African Americans during the transition to adulthood. *Journal of Youth and Adolescence,* 38(2), 242–57.

Hartmann, H. (2003). Closing the gap amidst ongoing discrimination: Women and economic disparities. *Multinational Monitor,* 24(5), 25–27.

Heflinger, C. A., and Christens, B. (2006). Rural behavioral health services for children and adolescents: An ecological and community psychology analysis. *Journal of Community Psychology,* 34, 379–400.

Henry, M. (2007). If the shoe fits: Authenticity, authority and agency feminist diasporic research. *Women's Studies International Forum,* 30, 70–80.

Herman-Stahl, M., Ashley, O., Penne, M., and Bauman, K. (2007). Serious psychological distress among parenting and nonparenting adults. *American Journal of Public Health,* 97(12), 2222–29.

Hirschmann, N. J. (2003). *The subject of liberty: Toward a feminist theory of freedom.* Princeton, NJ: Princeton University Press.

Hubbard, R. L., Craddock, S. G., Flynn, P. M., Anderson, J., and Etheridge, R. M. (1997). Overview of 1-year follow-up outcomes in the Drug Abuse Treatment Outcome Study (DATOS). *Psychology of Addictive Behaviors,* 11(4), 261–78.

Inciardi, J. A., and Surratt, H. L. (2001). Drug use, street crime, and sex-trading among cocaine-dependent women: Implications for public health and criminal justice policy. *Journal of Psychoactive Drugs,* 33, 379–89.

James, S., Johnson, J., Raghavan, C., and Lemos, T. (2003). The violent matrix: A study of structural, interpersonal, and intrapersonal violence among a sample of poor women. *American Journal of Community Psychology,* 31(1/2), 129–44.

Kasper, J. D., Ensminger, M. E., Green, K. M., Fothergill, K. E., Juon, H-S., Robertson, J., and Thorpe, R. J. (2008). Effects of poverty and family stress over three decades on the functional status of older African American women. *Journals of Gerontology,* 63B(4), S201–10.

Kelly, B. D. (2006). The power gap: freedom, power and mental illness. *Social Science and Medicine,* 63(8), 2118–26.

Kemmis, S., and McTaggart, R. (2000). Participatory action research. In N. K. Denzin and Y. S. Lincoln (Eds.), *The handbook of qualitative research.* Thousand Oaks, CA: Sage Publications. 567–605.

Kempadoo, K., and Doezma, J. (1998). *Global sex workers: Rights, resistance and redefinition.* London: Routledge.

Kinnell, H. (2006). Murder made easy: the final solution to prostitution? In

M. O'Neill and R. Campbell (Eds.), *Sex Work Now*. Cullumpton, UK: Willan Press. 141–68.

Kittay, E. F. (1998). Welfare, dependency, and a public ethics of care. *Social Justice, 25*(1), 123–45.

Kittay, E. F. (2001). A feminist public ethic of care meets the new communitarian family policy. *Ethics, 111*(3), 523–47.

Kleinman, A. (1988). *The illness narratives: Suffering, healing and the human condition.* New York: Basic Books.

Kleinman, A., Das, V., and Lock, M. (1997). *Social suffering.* Berkeley: University of California Press.

Kondrat, D., and Teater, B. (2009). An anti-stigma approach of working with persons with severe mental disability: Seeking real change through narrative change. *Journal of Social Work Practice, 23*(1), 35–47.

Koski-Jännes, A. (2004). In search of a comprehensive model of addiction. In P. Rosenqvist, J. Blomqvist, A. Koski-Jännes, and L. Öjesjö (Eds.), *Addiction and lifecourse.* Helsinki: NAD Publication 44. 49–67.

Kuno, E., and Rothbard, A. B. 2005. The effect of income and race on quality of psychiatric care in community mental health centers. *Community Mental Health Journal, 41* (5), 613–22.

Langer, G., Arnedt, C., and Sussman, D. (2004). Primetime live poll: American sex survey. *ABC News.* Retrieved July 16, 2008, from *abcnews.go.com/Primetime/PollVault/.*

Lazear, K., Pires, S., Isaacs, M., and Chaulk, P. (2008). Depression among low-income women of color: Qualitative findings from cross-cultural focus groups. *Journal of Immigrant and Minority Health, 10*(2), 127–33.

Marcel, G. (1951). *The mystery of being, vol. 1: Reflection and mystery.* G. S. Fraser, trans. London: Harvill Press.

May, G. G. (2007). *Addiction and grace: Love and spirituality in the healing of addictions.* New York: Harper One.

McFague, S. (2001). *Life abundant: Rethinking theology and economy for a planet in peril.* Minneapolis: Augsburg Fortress.

McKeganey, N. P., and McIntosh, J. (2000). *Drug misuse research in Scotland: The contribution of research to Scotland's drug misuse strategy.* Edinburgh: Scottish Executive: Effective Interventions Unit.

McKnight, J. (1995). *The careless society: Community and its counterfeits.* New York: Basic Books.

Melrose, M. (2007). The government's new prostitution strategy: A cheap fix for drug-using sex workers? *Community Safety Journal, 6*(1), 18–26.

Milio, J., Peltier, M. J., and Hufnail, M. (Executive Producers). (2000). *His-*

tory of prostitution: Sex in the city [Television broadcast]. In *History's mysteries*. New York: History Channel.

Morrison, N., and Severino, S. (2009). *Sacred desire: Growing in compassionate living*. West Conshohocken, PA: Templeton Foundation Press.

Mulia, N. (2000). Questioning sex: Drug-using women and heterosexual relations. *Journal of Drug Issues*, 30(4), 741–66.

Mulia, N. (2002). Ironies in the pursuit of well-being: The perspectives of low-income, substance-using women on service institutions. *Contemporary Drug Problems*, 29(4), 711–48.

Nagar, R. (2002). Footloose researchers, traveling theories and the politics of transnational feminist praxis. *Gender, Place and Culture*, 9(2), 179–86.

Nagle, J. (1997). *Whores and other feminists*. New York: Routledge.

Nandon, S. M., Koverola, C., and Schludermann, E. (1998). Antecedents to prostitution: Childhood victimization. *Journal of Interpersonal Violence*, 206(16).

National Institute of Justice. (1998). *Annual Report of Adult and Juvenile Arrestees* (NCJ Publication 171672). Washington, DC: US Department of Justice.

Nussbaum, M. (1999). *Sex and social justice*. Oxford: Oxford University Press.

Nussbaum, M. (2000). *Women and human development: The capabilities approach*. Cambridge: Cambridge University Press.

Nuttbrock, L. A. (2004). Linking female sex workers with substance abuse treatment. *Journal of Substance Abuse Treatment*, 27, 235–39.

O'Neill, M. (2001). *Prostitution and feminism: Towards a politics of feeling*. Cambridge, UK: Polity Press.

O'Neill, M. (2007). Community, safety, rights and recognition: Towards a coordinated prostitution strategy? *Community Safety Journal*, 6(1), 45–52.

Pargament, K. (2007). *Spiritually integrated psychotherapy: Understanding and addressing the sacred*. New York: Guilford Press.

Parpart, J. (2002). Lessons from the field: Rethinking empowerment, gender and development from a post- (post-?) development perspective. In K. Saunders (Ed.), *Feminist post-development thought: Rethinking modernity, post-colonialism and representation*. London: Zed Books. 41–55.

Pateman, C. (1988). *The sexual contract*. Stanford, CA: Stanford University Press.

Petro, M. (2007). "I did it . . . for the money": Sex work as a means to socio-economic opportunity. *Research for Sex Work, No. 9*. Retrieved December 12, 2007, from *www.nswp.org*.

Phelan, J., Yang, L., and Cruz-Rojas, R. (2006). Effects of attributing serious mental illnesses to genetic causes on orientations to treatment. *Psychiatric Services, 57*(3), 382–87.

Polletta, Francesca (2006). *It was like a fever: Storytelling in protest and politics.* Chicago: University of Chicago Press.

Prilleltensky, I., and Nelson, G. (2002). *Doing psychology critically: Making a difference in diverse settings.* New York: Palgrave Macmillan.

ProCon.org. (2008). *Prostitution.* Retrieved August 8, 2008, from *prostitution. procon.org.*

Prussing, E. (2007). Reconfiguring the empty center: Drinking, sobriety and identity in Native American women's narratives. *Culture, Medicine and Psychiatry, 31*(4), 499–526.

Rafalovich, A. (1999). Keep coming back! Narcotics Anonymous narrative and recovering-addict identity. *Contemporary Drug Problems, 26*(1), 131–57.

Rappaport, J. (1995). Empowerment meets narrative: Listening to stories and creating settings. *American Journal of Community Psychology, 23*(5), 795–808.

Rappaport, J. (2000). Community narratives: Tales of terror and joy. *American Journal of Community Psychology, 28*(1), 1–24.

Ringdal, N. J. (1997). *Love for sale: A world history of prostitution.* New York: Grove Press.

Roberts, A., Jackson, M. S., and Carlton-LaNey, I. (2000). Revisiting the need for feminism and Afrocentric theory when treating African-American female substance abusers. *Journal of Drug Issues, 30*(4), 901–18.

Rochon, T. R. (2000). *Culture moves: Ideas, activism and changing values.* Princeton, NJ: Princeton University Press.

SAMHSA. (2006). *Therapeutic community curriculum* (DHHS Publication No. SMA 06-4122). Rockville, MD: Substance Abuse and Mental Health Services Administration.

SAMHSA. (2009). *Results from the 2008 National Survey on Drug Use and Health: National findings* (Office of Applied Studies, NSDUH Series H–36, HHS Publication No. SMA 09-4434). Rockville, MD: Substance Abuse and Mental Health Services Administration.

Sanders, T., and Campbell, R. (2007). Designing out vulnerability, building in respect: Violence, safety and sex work policy. *British Journal of Sociology, 58*(1), 1–19.

Sen, A. (1999). *Development as freedom.* New York: First Anchor Books.

Shaffer, K., and Smith, S. (2004). *Human rights and narrated lives: The ethics of recognition.* New York: Palgrave Macmillan.

Shuman, J., and Meador, K. (2003). *Heal thyself: Spirituality, medicine, and the distortion of Christianity*. New York: Oxford University Press.

Singer, M. (2008). *Drugging the poor: Legal and illegal drugs and social inequality*. Long Grove, IL: Waveland Press.

Singh, J. P., and Hart, S. A. (2007). Sex workers and cultural policy: Mapping the issues and actors in Thailand. *Review of Policy Research, 24*(2), 155–73.

Smedley, B., Stith, A., and Nelson, A. (Eds.) (2004). *Unequal treatment: Confronting racial and ethnic disparities in health care*. Washington, DC: Institute of Medicine, National Academies Press.

Snarr, C. M. (2007). *Social selves and political reform: Five visions in contemporary Christian ethics*. New York: T. and T. Clark.

Spivak, G. (1988). Can the subaltern speak? In C. Nelson and L. Grossberg (Eds.), *Marxism and the interpretation of cultures*. Urbana: University of Illinois Press. 271–315.

Stevens, B. (2008). Introduction and invitation. In Women of Magdalene, with Becca Stevens, *Find your way home: Words from the street, wisdom from the heart*. Nashville: Abingdon Press.

Stolz, J., Shannon, K., Kerr, T., Zhang, R., Motaner, J., and Wood, E. (2007). Associations between childhood maltreatment and sex work in a cohort of drug-using youth. *Social Science and Medicine, 65*, 1214–21

Surratt, H., Inciardi, J., Kurtz, S., and Kiley, M. (2004). Sex work and drug use in a subculture of violence. *Crime and Delinquency 50*(1), 43–59.

Tennessee Housing Development Agency. (2009). *Tennessee housing at a glance*. Retrieved March 24, 2009, from *www.thda.org/news/hsgglance08.pdf*.

Thistle Farms. (2008). *www.thistlefarms.org*. Retrieved August 8, 2008.

Tronto, Joan. (1993). *Moral boundaries: A political argument for an ethic of care*. New York: Routledge, Chapman and Hall.

US Census Bureau. (2008). *American community survey: Selected economic characteristics, 2005–2009* [data]. Retrieved May 15, 2009, from *factfinder.census.gov/*.

USD HHS (US Department of Health and Human Services, Administration on Children, Youth and Families). (2007). *Child maltreatment 2007*. Washington, DC: GPO. Retrieved April 4, 2010, from *www.acf.hhs.gov/programs/cb*.

USD HUD (US Department of Housing and Urban Development). (2009). *The 2008 annual homelessness assessment report to Congress*. Retrieved April 4, 2010, from *www.hmis.info/classicAsp/documents/2008AHARSummary.pdf*.

Vaddiparti, K., Bogetto, J., Callahan, C., Abdallah, A., Spitznagel, E., and Cottler, L. (2006). The effects of childhood trauma on sex trading in substance using women. *Archives of Sexual Behavior, 35,* 451–59.

Vanwesenbeeck, I. (2001). Another decade of social scientific sex work: A review of research 1900–2000. *Annual Review of Sex Research, 12,* 242–89.

Wang, P. S., Lane, M., Olfson, M., Pincus, H. A., Wells, K. B., and Kessler, R. C. (2005). Twelve-month use of mental health services in the United States: Results from the National Comorbidity Survey Replication. *Archives of General Psychiatry 62,* 629–40.

Ward, H., Day, S., and Weber, J. (1999). Risky business: Health and safety in the sex industry over a 9-year period. *Sexually Transmitted Infections, 7,* 340–43.

Weiss, R. (1994). *Learning from strangers: The art and method of qualitative interview studies.* New York: Free Press.

West, C. M., Williams, L. M., and Siegel, J. A. (2000). Adult sexual revictimization among black women sexually abused in childhood: A prospective examination of serious consequences of abuse. *Child Maltreatment, 5*(1), 49–67.

Wirzba, N. K. (2006). *Living the Sabbath: Discovering the rhythms of rest and delight.* Grand Rapids, MI: Brazos Press.

Women of Magdalene, with Becca Stevens. (2008). *Find your way home: Words from the street, wisdom from the heart.* Nashville: Abingdon Press.

Young, Michael P. (2007). *Bearing witness against sin: The evangelical birth of the American social movement.* Chicago: University of Chicago Press.

Zerai, A., and Banks, R. (2002). African American mothers' substance abuse: Punishment over treatment. *SIECUS Report, 30*(3), 26–29.

Zierler, S., and Feingold, L. (1991). Adult survivors of child sexual abuse and subsequent risk of HIV infection. *American Journal of Public Health, 81*(5), 572.

INDEX